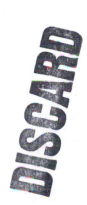

DISCARD

DEC - " 2005

DEMCO

Cataracts

A PATIENT'S GUIDE TO TREATMENT

David F. Chang, M.D. • Howard Gimbel, M.D.

Addicus Books
Omaha, Nebraska

An Addicus Nonfiction Book

ISBN# 1-886039-66-6
Cover design by George Foster
Illustrations by Jack Kusler and Bob Hogenmiller

This book is not intended to serve as a substitute for a physician. Nor is it the authors' intent to give medical advice contrary to that of an attending physician.

Library of Congress Cataloging-in-Publication Data
Chang, David, 1954-
  Cataracts : a patient's guide to treatment / David Chang, Howard Gimbel.
    p. cm.
  ISBN 1-886039-66-6 (alk. paper)
  1. Cataract—Surgery. 2. Patient education. I. Gimbel, Howard V., 1934- II. Title.
RE451.C43 2004
617.7'42059—dc22   2003025532

Addicus Books, Inc.
P.O. Box 45327
Omaha, Nebraska 68145
Web site: http://www.AddicusBooks.com

Printed in the United States of America
10 9 8 7 6 5 4 3 2 1

*To my dedicated staff, with gratitude for their daily,
tireless efforts in helping to educate and care for our patients.*
—D.C.

*To my wife Judy, who has always been
and continues to be my inspiration and support.*
—H.G.

v

Contents

Acknowledgments

I wish to acknowledge my office staff, some of whom have worked in our office for thirty years for their help in caring for my cataract patients. I would especially like to thank Sharon, Sue, Tera, Margita, Kaylin, Jeff, Sheri, Dianne, Karen, and Leslie.

I would also like to thank the hardworking and professional staff of Addicus Books, particularly Rod Colvin and Susan Adams, for their help in editing the text. Finally, I would like to thank my family for their patience in allowing me the time to write this book.

David Chang, M.D.

I would like to thank all those of my staff who have shared my passion for patient, family, and community education. This includes not only nurses and ophthalmic technicians, but also administrative and audiovisual staff members who help prepare and update educational materials.

I also wish to thank my wife and family who have been gracious in sharing our evening and weekend time to allow me time for writing and editing these chapters.

Howard Gimbel, M.D.

Introduction

If you have picked up this book, perhaps you're worried that you have a cataract. Maybe your vision has become blurry, or you feel as if you're looking through mist or a lace certain. You may find yourself backing away from some of your favorite activities, such as reading and work or hobbies, that require good vision. Perhaps you have difficulty seeing when you're driving at night. If you are experiencing such vision problems, you may have a cataract—one of the most common vision problems in North America.

The good news is that cataract surgery can restore your vision. Because we know that the thought surgery on your eyes may make you feel anxious, we have written this book to help you understand cataracts and allay your concerns. We will explain how cataracts form, how they're diagnosed, and how they are treated. We will also discuss follow-up care and special conditions that may affect cataract surgery. We believe that with this knowledge, you'll be better equipped to talk with your doctor about the best way to improve your vision. It is important that you be able to make an informed decision about cataract treatment that could make your world bright and clear once again.

Nothing in life is to be feared.
It is only to be understood.
—Marie Curie
1867-1934

1

How the Human Eye Works

"I just don't see as well as I used to."

You've probably said these words in frustration as you tried to thread a needle or hammer a nail. Maybe you've given up driving at night or surfing the Internet. Reading might not be as enjoyable as it once was. It might seem as though you continually need new eyeglass or contact lens prescriptions.

Of course, you're concerned. Of all our senses, *sight* may be the one we most rely on. We depend on our eyes for the ability to move about freely—to walk, drive, dance, or roller skate. Our eyes keep us mobile and independent. When your eyes transmit images to the brain, they supply a perpetual stream of information from the world around you.

Anatomy of the Eye

You've probably heard it said that the eye works much like a camera. It focuses light to form images, and then converts those images into nerve impulses for the brain to interpret. This is similar to the way a camera lens transmits images to film.

The eyes are spheres about an inch in diameter—self-lubricating, self-cleansing, well protected, and so sensitive that they can distinguish between images only one ten-thousandth of an inch apart. An eyeball is made up of several complex structures.

The *sclera* forms the round wall of the eyeball, the part we commonly refer to as the white of the eye. The sclera is a tough, thick, opaque structure that protects the delicate structures inside the eyeball. The *conjunctiva* is a thin mucous membrane that covers the sclera; this membrane, along with the eyelids, protects your eyeball from environmental irritants.

The *cornea* is a transparent, dome-like window at the front of the eye. As light enters your eye, the cornea bends, or refracts, the light before it passes through the lens. Unlike most other structures in your body, the cornea contains no blood vessels; instead, it receives oxygen from the air and other nourishment from the *aqueous humor*, a clear liquid between the cornea and lens. (The aqueous humor also keeps your eyeball inflated at the proper pressure.) Because it is rich in nerve fibers, the cornea is very sensitive. This is why you feel even the tiniest foreign object, such as dust or an eyelash, when it lands on your eye's surface.

The *iris* is the part of the eye we refer to when we describe the color of someone's eyes. Typically a shade of brown or blue,

Eyeball Anatomy

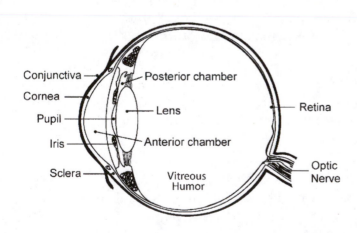

Conjunctiva — Posterior chamber
Cornea
Pupil — Lens — Retina
Iris — Anterior chamber
Sclera — Vitreous Humor — Optic Nerve

the iris sits behind the cornea and acts like a curtain as it controls the amount of light entering the eye.

The *pupil* is the black hole in the center of your iris that determines the amount of light entering the eye. In low light, the muscles of the iris cause the pupil to open wide or dilate; likewise, the pupil constricts in bright light.

The *lens,* which sits just behind the pupil, is really a flexible bag of clear protein that helps focus light onto your retina. Surrounded by a thin membrane called the *capsule* or *capsular bag,* the lens is shaped like a piece of M&M candy. It

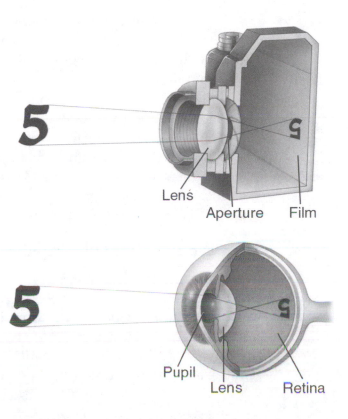

The above illustration demonstrates the similarities between a camera and the eyeball. Courtesy American Academy of Ophthalmology

changes shape—flattening or thickening to bring objects at various distances into focus—in a process called *accommodation.* The lens loses flexibility over time, and by our early forties most of us find that it's harder for our eyes to shift focus.

The *retina* lines the back half of your eyeball. About the size of a postage stamp and as thin as onion skin, the retina is the "film" of the camera. It registers light images and sends them to your brain through a bundle of nerve fibers called the *optic nerve.* Your brain then "develops the film," interpreting the shapes, colors, and details of the images it receives.

The cavity between the lens and the retina is filled with a transparent gel-like substance called the *vitreous humor,* through which light rays pass from the lens to your retina. As this gel becomes more watery with age, tiny residual solid portions can move. This creates harmless drifting shadows known as *floaters.*

How the Eyes Stay Lubricated

The surface of your eye is constantly lubricated by a steady production of *tears,* a marvelous process provided by nature. Tears flow from glands at the outer, upper corners of the eyes, and drain through tiny tear ducts in the inner corners of our upper and lower eyelids. When we blink, we pump tears from the eye surface into the tear duct drainage system. This is why if we are about to cry, we start to blink more as our eyes are welling up with tears. Rapid blinking pumps the tears into the tear ducts.

The tear ducts pass through channels within the bones of the nose and eventually empty the tears into the back of your throat. This also explains the otherwise puzzling phenomenon of being able to taste eyedrops.

Americans with Vision Problems

Refractive error	150 million
Cataracts	20.5 million
Diabetic retinopathy	5.3 million
Glaucoma	2.2 million
Macular degeneration	1.6 million

Source: Prevent Blindness America

Common Vision Problems

Refractive Errors

There are two basic causes of blurred vision: refractive error and eye disease. Refractive errors are common, natural optical imperfections that are easily treated with glasses or contact lenses. Four common examples are described below.

Nearsightedness (myopia) occurs when the eye bends light too soon, focusing the rays in front of rather than on the retina. If you are myopic, you see nearby objects better than you see faraway ones. Images in the distance appear blurry.

Farsightedness (hyperopia) occurs when the eye bends light too late, focusing the rays behind the retina. If you're farsighted, both far and near images appear blurry, but the closer the object, the blurrier it is.

Presbyopia is a result of normal age-related changes in the lens, which becomes less flexible over time. As the lens stiffens, the eye

Normal Vision

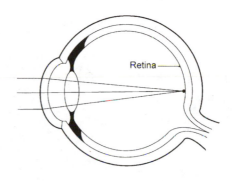

When one has normal vision, light rays enter through the cornea and lens and strike the retina, producing a focused image.

Myopia

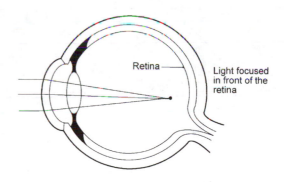

In myopia, nearsightedness, light rays focus in front of the retina, causing distant objects to appear blurry.

Hyperopia

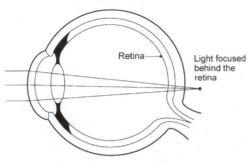

With hyperopia, farsightedness, light rays focus behind the retina. Objects in the distance are seen less blurry than near objects.

Astigmatism

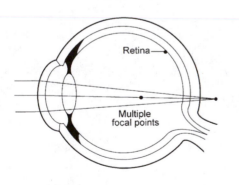

In astigmatism, light entering the eyeball focuses on multiple areas rather than on the retina. Objects both far and near appear blurry.

muscles responsible for accommodation can no longer change the lens shape enough for you to focus on close objects. If you're in your forties or older, you've probably experienced this unavoidable condition. You may have started wearing reading glasses or bifocals.

Astigmatism occurs when the cornea's curvature is oblong like the back of a spoon, instead of rounded like a basketball. This common condition causes blurred vision for objects both near and far.

Common Eye Disorders

The second category of conditions impairing vision consists of abnormalities not correctable with glasses because they involve the vision-producing structures of the eye. Cataracts are one such condition; others are briefly introduced below and discussed in more detail in Chapter Nine.

Macular degeneration is one of a dozen or so conditions that can affect the retina. A painless disorder common among older people, macular degeneration is caused by age-related deterioration of the central part of the retina, the *macula*. Macular degeneration may cause a gradual deterioration of central vision. Although it is a potentially serious problem, the vast majority of patients will not suffer severe vision loss. There is a wide spectrum in the severity of the problem.

Glaucoma, which also occurs more often as we age, is a condition in which the pressure of the fluid in the eye becomes too high. If diagnosed early enough, glaucoma can be treated with eyedrop medications that lower the fluid pressure. Left untreated, glaucoma can ruin the optic nerve and lead to blindness.

Diabetic retinopathy refers to circulation problems in the retina that results from years of elevated blood sugar. Fluid may leak out of diseased blood vessels into the retina, or abnormal vessels in the retina may bleed into the vitreous cavity. Although laser treatments or surgery can help, the best course is prevention through consistent control of blood sugar levels.

Other health conditions can cause blurry vision, so don't delay seeing your doctor if you experience a reduction in the clarity of your vision. The right diagnosis and proper treatment can protect your eyes and preserve—or improve—your vision.

2

Understanding Cataracts

If you've reached your sixties, you probably have begun to feel some of the effects of aging on your vision. Most of us are not seeing as well as we once did, and cataracts may be a factor. In fact, for those over age 40, cataracts are one of the most common reasons for poor eyesight. Cataracts are the most common cause of reversible vision loss in North America. In developing countries where cataract surgery is often unavailable, cataracts are the leading cause of blindness.

Most cataracts are the result of aging. These cataracts often begin in one's forties or fifties, but they may not affect vision until after age 60. According to the American Academy of Ophthalmology, between the ages of 52 and 64, you have a 50–50 chance of developing a cataract. By age 75, nearly everyone has at least some cataract formation.

What Is a Cataract?

The word *cataract* comes from the Greek word for waterfall. It was once believed that a milky substance "falling" into the eye caused cataracts. Today, we know that a cataract is a gradual clouding of the eye's lens. How does this come about? The lens is made mostly of protein and water. Sometimes the nature of the protein can change, creating a cloudiness in areas of the lens. As a result, light does not pass through the lens as well and vision is affected.

There is often confusion about the definition of the word cataract. A cataract is not a growth on the lens. A cataract is the clouded lens itself.

Types of Cataracts

There are several basic types of cataracts. It is important to note that the type or location is not as important as the severity of a cataract. The severity, whether it is mild, moderate, or advanced, determines the need for corrective surgery. The type of cataract has no real bearing on the need for surgery.

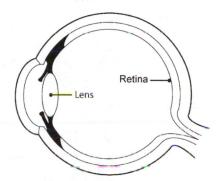

The normal eyeball has a clear lens through which light can pass.

- *Age-related* cataracts form as the eyeball ages.
- *Traumatic* cataracts develop after an eye injury (may be years later).
- *Congenital* cataracts appear in babies or develop in children, often in both eyes.

Cataracts can also be classified according to their location within the lens. *Nuclear cataracts,* the most common, form in the center of the

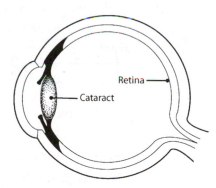

In this eye, a cataract has formed. Note how lens has become cloudy.

9

lens. *Cortical cataracts* are spokelike, beginning near the outer part of the lens and extending inward toward the center. *Subcapsular cataracts* begin at the front or back of the lens; they often develop slowly, but sometimes develop very quickly.

Symptoms of Cataracts

How do you know if you have cataracts? They usually can't be seen with the naked eye. They're painless, their progress is typically gradual, and they don't cause symptoms such as redness or tearing. The loss of visual acuity, or sharpness, in one or both eyes is progressive, but slow. Consequently, many people don't even realize they have cataracts at first. Individual symptoms vary greatly, depending on the severity, location, and type of cataract. Some people experience a loss of contrast in colors and occasionally may experience double vision in one eye with cataracts. Others have trouble seeing in dim light. Some may notice a troublesome glare in bright sunlight or when facing oncoming headlights in traffic.

What are some indications that you may have cataracts? If you answer "yes" to several of the following questions, you may have cataracts:

- Is your vision blurry, cloudy, or foggy?
- Do you have trouble seeing distant details, such as highway signs?
- Do you need more light for close work?
- Do your eyes tire more easily when reading?
- Do you have trouble seeing in restaurants and other dimly lit rooms?

- Is your night vision poor?
- Does glare bother you, making it harder for you to drive at night or to see well in bright sunlight?
- Do you see ghost images, such as two or three moons at night?
- Do colors appear faded, washed out, or yellowish?
- Does your eyeglass prescription change more frequently as your nearsightedness becomes more severe?

It is a common misconception that cataracts are visible to the naked eye. In fact, people often mistake whitish growths on the surface of the eye for cataracts, when that is not the case. Usually these are callous-like growths that result from the cumulative effect of irritation caused by dryness and sunlight over many years. Similarly, as we age, we may develop a hazy white ring around the edges of the cornea. Many people think these rings are cataracts, but they are actually an accumulation of cholesterol, deposited by nearby blood vessels. They do not affect vision and do not represent an abnormal cholesterol level. They simply are a sign of aging. Like gray hair, they have no real health significance.

How Cataracts Progress

In the early stages, cataracts may not cause vision problems. The cloudiness may affect only a small portion of the lens. However, over time the cloudiness increases, making vision worse. The speed with which they progress varies greatly with each person. Some individuals may not notice symptoms for years. In other cases, vision deteriorates more rapidly. In rare cases, cataracts progress after only a few months.

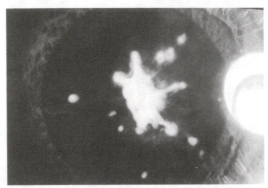

This cataract resembles a splotch of mud. The round glow at the right of the picture is a reflection from the light used in the eye exam.

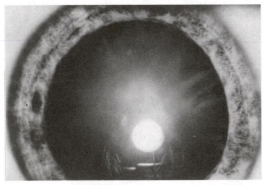

This age-related cataract is more diffuse or scattered. Note how it appears as a haze throughout the lens.

It is impossible to predict when you will need surgery. Once vision begins to deteriorate quickly, the need for surgery becomes quite obvious. Because cataracts are a result of normal aging, they eventually develop in both eyes. It's not uncommon for one eye to develop a cataract earlier or more quickly than the other. This doesn't mean that the eye with the worse cataract is abnormal or in poorer health than the other eye. A cataract in one eye does not affect the health or function of the other eye.

Other than lens clouding, cataracts do not damage or harm your eyes. So the decision to have surgery is based primarily on your symptoms and the dègree to which they interfere with your day-to-day life. If you're having no trouble with normal activities and you're satisfied with your eyesight, there's no pressing need to have a cataract removed.

As the cataract progresses, the lens becomes cloudier and eventually opaque. If it is not removed, the cataract can eventually obscure all useful vision in the affected eye. This does not happen all at once, but rather occurs in stages (except in the case of traumatic cataracts that form soon after a severe eye injury). The most advanced cataracts, called *mature,* cause the entire lens to turn white. At this point, the eye is functionally blind. If your cataract is already very advanced, don't wait for it to become this severe before having it removed.

Causes and Risk Factors

Scientists don't know the precise biological mechanisms that cause cataracts. However, they are exploring the theory that age-related cataracts develop when certain eye proteins, called *alpha-crystallins*, fail as the eyes get older. Alpha-crystallins do the important work of protecting lens proteins; without them, the normally clear lens proteins would clump and lose their transparency. But like other body cells, alpha-crystallins can be damaged by so-called *free radicals* (also called oxygenating agents). Free radicals are highly charged, highly unstable molecule fragments that harm healthy cells. Over time, damage from free radicals may prevent alpha-crystallins from doing their protective job, and cataracts develop.

As mentioned, age is the greatest risk factor related to the onset of cataracts. Cataracts are the most common cause of blurred vision in people over age 50. There are several other risk factors which you also generally have no control over, including:

- **Family history.** In certain families, cataracts tend to occur at earlier ages. Knowing at what age your parents developed cataracts, however, doesn't necessarily tell you at what age you might expect them.

- **Medical disorders.** Being diabetic raises the risk of cataracts three- to four-fold. High blood sugar levels react with proteins in the eye, forming by-products that accumulate in the lens. Treatments for some illnesses, such as radiation to the head and total-body radiation treatments for cancer, can also induce cataracts. Rarely do cataracts occur at birth or develop during early childhood but when they do, the cause is usually unknown. However, diseases, inherited disorders, and infections during pregnancy (such as rubella) can play a part.

- **Race.** Native Americans and African Americans are at higher risk than Caucasians for cataracts.

- **Nearsightedness.** People with more severe myopia can develop cataracts at an earlier age and may need surgery by the time they are in their forties or fifties.

- **Steroid use.** If you take systemic steroid medications over a long period of time for conditions such as asthma or emphysema, you're at increased risk for cataracts. Long-term use of high doses of inhaled steroids also increases the risk. This is not true of lower doses.

- **Eye diseases.** Certain eye diseases such as chronic internal eye inflammation, called uveitis or iritis, are associated with cataracts. Some babies born prematurely develop a retinal disease during infancy, called retinopathy of prematurity. They are prone to developing cataracts in their forties.

- **Eye injuries.** Severe trauma to the eyes at any age can cause cataracts to develop, even many years later. Cataracts can be caused by sharp objects or metal particles that penetrate the eye or by blunt injuries, such as the impact from a ball, a punch, or a firecracker explosion. Eye injuries are the leading cause of cataracts in children and adolescents.

Preventing Cataracts

Several large studies have looked at whether certain vitamin or mineral supplements can prevent or delay cataracts. Unfortunately, the results have been disappointing. One landmark study showed that antioxidants have no effect on preventing cataracts. Other studies show that certain medications and eyedrops, touted as preventing cataracts, are also ineffective.

You can, however, take some steps that may *delay* the progression of cataracts and protect your overall health, as well:

- **Don't smoke.** Cataracts occur more frequently among smokers. The evidence is clear: stop smoking. It is the single most important thing you can do to prevent cataracts.
- **Eat fruits and vegetables.** There is some evidence that a diet with plenty of fruits and vegetables may delay the onset of cataracts.
- **Protect your eyes from excessive sun exposure.** A hat with a brim can reduce sunlight exposure to your eyes by 30 to 50 percent. Wear sunglasses outdoors and protective eye goggles in tanning booths.

- **Manage diabetes well.** Work with your doctor to keep your blood sugar under control.
- **Avoid eye injuries.** Wear protective goggles when performing tasks that could result in eye injury. According to the United States Eye Injury Registry, 40 percent of eye injuries occur in the home, 13 percent occur in industrial settings, and 13 percent occur during sporting activities. Blunt objects account for 31 percent of injuries. Sharp objects cause 18 percent of eye injuries. Other causes include vehicle crashes, BB and pellet guns, nails, hammer on metal, fireworks, guns, falls, and explosions.

3

Getting a Diagnosis

In the early stages of cataracts, vision problems may not interfere with your everyday activities such as reading, driving, or watching television. And at first, you may be able to compensate for your vision loss by using different eyeglasses, a magnifying glass, or stronger lighting. However, as cataracts progress, vision problems become worse. Accordingly, it is important to get a diagnosis.

Role of Eye Care Specialists

Ophthalmologists

Several types of health professionals are involved in eye care. An *ophthalmologist* is a medical doctor who specializes in medical and surgical eye care. *General ophthalmologists* diagnose and treat eye problems, including common conditions that require surgery, such as cataracts. They also perform vision examinations and prescribe eyeglasses and contact lenses. *Specialist ophthalmologists* undergo additional training and choose to specialize in surgery and treatment of a particular part of the eye; for example, they may be retina specialists or cornea specialists.

Ophthalmologists have extensive training and education—at least four years of pre-medical college education, four or more years of medical school, a one-year internship, and three or more years of specialized medical and surgical training in eye diseases.

Optometrists

Optometrists are licensed to provide basic eye care services, including testing for vision problems such as nearsightedness or farsightedness. They also diagnose eye conditions and diseases such as cataracts. These eye doctors also prescribe corrective lenses (glasses and contacts) and medications for some eye disorders. Optometrists do not perform surgery, but they may advise you about surgery. For example, your optometrist can diagnose your cataracts and help you decide when you should consider having cataract surgery. He or she can also refer you to a qualified ophthalmologist for surgery.

Optometrists complete two to four years of undergraduate studies and four years of postgraduate optometry school.

Opticians

Although *opticians* are not involved with the diagnosis of cataracts or other diseases, it may be helpful to clarify the role they play in your eye care. Opticians design, finish, fit, and dispense eyeglasses and contact lenses, based on an eye doctor's prescription. Opticians may also dispense colored and specialty contact lenses for special needs.

Your Appointment with an Eye Doctor

When you go to an eye specialist, he or she will perform a thorough examination, including a microscopic examination of the interior of your eyeballs. He or she will also use viewing instruments to discover if cataracts are present. During the exam, the doctor will ask questions about your eye history. This examination will be painless and can uncover other preventable or treatable problems that might damage your vision. During a complete eye exam, your doctor will:

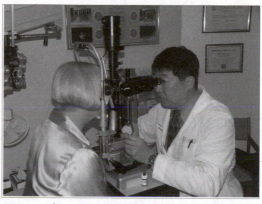

Here a doctor uses a special microscope, called a slit lamp, to examine a patient's eye lens for possible cataracts.

- Take your eye medical history
- Give you a vision test and check your eyeglass prescription
- Examine the exterior of your eyeballs
- Examine the interior of your eyeballs
- Measure the fluid pressure within the eyeball

Your Eye and Medical History

Your doctor will want to know about any eye symptoms you are having. Try to be as accurate as possible in describing your symptoms. If your vision is impaired, explain which activities are difficult.

Your eye doctor will ask about your eye history and want to know when you had your last eye exam. You should mention any previous eye diseases, injuries, or surgeries you have had. List any prescription eye medications that you are taking. Also tell your doctor if there is a history of glaucoma or retinal detachment in your family.

Your eye doctor needs to know about any major medical issues you may have. Common health problems such as diabetes, hypertension, heart disease, asthma, and emphysema can affect your eye health and impact your treatment decisions. Your doctor will want to know about any prescription medications you are taking, as well as allergies to medications.

Some medical problems can affect your comfort or your ability to cooperate during cataract surgery. Let your eye doctor know if you are hard of hearing, have claustrophobia, panic attacks, or sudden coughing attacks, or if you are allergic to latex. Also, let the doctor know if you have back pain, breathing problems or any other condition that might make it difficult for you to lie flat.

> *It is a common misconception that cataracts form on the surface of the eyes and they can be peeled off. However, the entire lens must be removed.*
> — Dr. Howard Gimbel

Assessing Your Vision

One of the first things your eye doctor will want to do during your eye exam is assess your vision. If you're having difficulty seeing, you may have a health problem with your eye or you may simply need glasses to correct your eye's inability to focus well. Your doctor will want to assess your eyesight using a standard eye chart.

What Is 20/20 Vision?

You've probably heard of 20/20 vision. But what exactly does it mean? This measure of visual acuity is based on how well you can read a vision chart from 20 feet away while you are wearing your glasses or contact lenses. The visual acuity chart, known as the Snellen Chart, contains twelve to thirteen rows of letters. The letters are largest in the top row and become progressively smaller with each descending row. Your visual acuity score is based on the smallest row of letters you are able to read.

Scores relate to how well someone with "perfect" vision reads the chart. For example, if your vision is 20/60 with your glasses on it means you read the chart at 20 feet as well as someone with perfect vision could read from 60 feet away.

Visual acuity can be tested with or without your eyeglasses. Your doctor will be more interested in your visual acuity score with your eyeglasses. Since healthy eyes should have excellent vision with the proper eyeglasses, testing your vision with your glasses on is the only way for your doctor to measure the effect of eye abnormalities such as cataracts and macular degeneration.

Although standard visual acuity tests are valuable, they do have limitations and do not address other vision problems cataracts may be causing. For example, the standard eye chart is not a good test for problems you may be having with contrast, color, glare, or peripheral vision.

> *Many people mistakenly believe that they must wait until a cataract is "ripe" before it can be surgically removed.*
>
> —Dr. David Chang

Determining Refractive Error

If you are having problems seeing well at different distances without glasses, it is important to determine whether you simply need new eyeglasses or whether you have another problem, such as a cataract. As part of your eye exam, your doctor will need to determine your refractive error. This refers to natural imperfections in the optics of the eye that reduce how sharply images are focused onto your retina.

Since your vision problem may be solved with new glasses, your doctor will want to first determine the best eyeglass prescription for each of your eyes. This process, called the *refraction*, identifies, measures, and quantifies the refractive error in each eye. The results of the refraction test will determine whether your lens prescription needs to be changed and, if so, by how much. Once your doctor has identified the best lens prescription for you, he or she will retest your ability to read the eye chart. If your vision is still abnormal, it indicates that you have a problem with the eye itself and further testing is needed.

Examining the Eyeball

Exterior of the Eyeball

During the examination of the exterior of your eye, your doctor will check the surface of the eye as well as the eyelids, looking for problems such as redness, irritation, swelling, scratches, or foreign bodies. He or she will also evaluate the movement of your eyes, both separately and together.

Your doctor will first examine the exterior surface of the eyeball with a *slit lamp*, a table-mounted microscope that allows the doctor to see both the surface and the interior of the eyeball with amazing detail. For instance, the slit lamp allows the doctor to see in three dimensions tiny individual blood vessels in the retina that are less than one-tenth of a millimeter wide.

In general, problems that involve the exterior surface of the eye usually do not affect vision. They can, however, cause discomfort and affect the appearance of your eye. For instance, a scratch on the surface of your cornea will cause a sharp pain every time you blink. Engorged surface blood vessels in the conjunctiva may cause your eyes to appear red or bloodshot. Other symptoms such as mucous, tearing, swelling, sharp pain, scratchiness, itching, and generalized discomfort usually reflect problems with the exterior surface of the eyeball. Examples of common and annoying conditions that affect the eye's exterior include dry eyes, misdirected eyelashes, styes and other lid problems, and conjunctivitis (pinkeye).

Interior of the Eyeball

It is during the examination of the interior of the eyeball that your doctor will determine whether you have a cataract. Prior to examining your eye interior, the doctor will dilate your pupil with eyedrops. Why is this important? The lens of the eye and other important structures are located behind the pupil. When light strikes our pupils, they constrict, or become smaller, making it difficult for the doctor to see inside the eyeball. The dilating drops temporarily inhibit this reaction. During the exam, the doctor will also use several illuminating and magnifying instruments, including the slit lamp, to examine the inside of your eyeball.

If you have a cataract, the slit lamp also makes it possible for the doctor to determine the characteristics of the cataract. Is the cataract *diffuse,* meaning the entire lens is cloudy? Or is the cataract *focal,* with the cloudiness appearing in patches? To better understand how a cataract may be forming, consider the analogy of dust on a car windshield. A layer of dust may cover the entire windshield, and it may be a light layer or quite thick; or splotches of dirt may appear on various parts of the windshield. Similarly, the cloudiness created by the cataract may take many shapes or forms.

While your pupil is dilated, the doctor will also check those structures that lie behind the iris and the lens, including the vitreous humor, retina, and optic nerve. Abnormalities with any of these structures could create vision problems.

When the pupil has been dilated, it allows more light than usual to enter the eye. While this is not harmful, you may feel uncomfortable in bright environments while your eyes are dilated. You may be more comfortable wearing sunglasses when you leave the doctor's office. The dilating drops wear off in several hours.

Measuring Eye Pressure

Another important part of the complete eye exam is the measurement of the eye's internal fluid pressure, or intraocular pressure. What is this fluid and why is the pressure important? It is a clear fluid called aqueous humor that circulates through the interior of the eyeball to keep it properly inflated.

As we age, the microscopic drainage area within the eye can clog. If fluid does not drain properly, pressure gradually increases. You can't feel this pressure; the amount of fluid is only about one-eighth teaspoon. However, over time the excessive fluid pressure can seriously damage the optic nerve. This condition is known as *glaucoma.* Once it is diagnosed, the high fluid pressure can be lowered with daily eyedrop medications.

Measuring the internal eye pressure with a glaucoma test is safe, simple, and painless. The doctor uses anesthetic eyedrops to numb the surface of the eyeball. He or she then uses a *tonometer,* a special pressure-sensing probe, usually mounted on the slit lamp microscope, to determine the pressure in the eyeball.

4

Your Intraocular Lens

Thanks to modern medicine, cataract treatment today involves an efficient surgical procedure during which the clouded lens is removed and a new, artificial lens is inserted into the eye. This lens is called an *intraocular lens*, or *IOL*, an artificial lens that is permanent. The development of the IOL was a remarkable achievement and represents one of the most important medical advances in the history of ophthalmology. Let's consider the history of cataract treatment and take a closer look at this incredible artificial lens—the lens that will restore your vision if you have cataracts.

Before IOLs: History of Cataract Treatment

Aphakia refers to the absence of a lens in the eye. The aphakic eye is functionally blind. Before the invention of intraocular lenses, there were two options for replacing the optical power of the extracted natural lens: aphakic spectacles and aphakic contact lenses.

Special glasses called *aphakic spectacles* or cataract glasses, were most commonly used to restore the focus after the cataract was removed. Because so much power had to be placed in the lenses, aphakic spectacles neither looked nor worked like conventional glasses. They were thick, heavy, uncomfortable, and

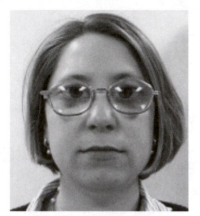

Prior to modern cataract surgery, patients wore aphakic glasses, which had thick, heavy lenses.

Photo courtesy Museum of Vision

unattractive. Furthermore, the unusually thick lenses magnified objects by approximately 25 percent. Although this worked fine for reading or other close work, it created unnatural visual distortions at other distances and made everyday activities like walking difficult. The aphakic spectacles also compromised depth perception and peripheral vision and created blind spots that caused images to suddenly pop in and out. Understandably, people had great difficulty adapting to them. Also, people who required cataract surgery in only one eye couldn't use them because the treated eye would see everything magnified, causing double vision. Aphakic spectacles are still used in some developing countries where artificial lenses and other modern medical technology are not available.

For those who could wear them, *aphakic contact lenses* were an improvement over aphakic spectacles. They provided the necessary optical power, but magnification with the contact lenses was negligible (less than 5 percent). As a result, they avoided the troublesome visual distortion of aphakic spectacles. For this reason, they could also be used following cataract surgery involving only one eye.

However, wearing aphakic contact lenses also posed problems. They could be uncomfortable for many older people. With age, the eye surface becomes drier and more prone to discomfort, which makes it harder for some individuals to wear contacts. Additionally, one must have good eyesight and good manual dexterity to be able to clean, handle, insert, and remove contact lenses.

If a patient had a contact lens fall out or get lost, he or she couldn't see at all with that eye. Unlike a nearsighted person who can see a contact lens on his or her fingertip, a person with aphakic eyes has extremely blurry near vision without contacts or glasses. This makes handling the contacts much more challenging than for nearsighted wearers. Although extended-wear contact lenses were often tried, serious infections were more common if the lenses were worn for longer than one week at a time.

In the past, people who had cataract surgery simply traded their poor vision for the visual distortion of aphakic glasses or the inconvenience of aphakic contacts. Because of such disadvantages, ophthalmologists often postponed cataract surgery until a person's

> *An IOL is a wonderful invention. Technology has provided us with more than 65 different lens powers to choose from.*
> —Dr. David Chang

cataract was more mature (advanced and hard). Then, even the distortion of aphakic spectacles after surgery would seem like a great improvement to the patient. This condition also made the surgery easier to perform with the surgical techniques available at the time.

Invention of the Intraocular Lens

During the Second World War, British ophthalmologist Harold Ridley treated several fighter pilots who had splinters from shattered aircraft canopies penetrating the interior of their eyeballs. To his amazement, Dr. Ridley found that, unlike other foreign materials that became lodged inside the eyeball following

Characteristics of Modern IOLs

- Permanently fixed inside the eye
- Made of a transparent material that should never cloud
- No moving parts that can wear out
- Lightweight and flexible
- Not affected by physical activities or by rubbing the eye
- Cannot be felt within the eye
- Provide the best possible vision correction
- Do not require cleaning
- Do not change the appearance or comfort of the eye
- Can be folded for insertion through a small incision; it then unfolds to original size

injuries, these pieces of plastic did not cause severe inflammation. Recognizing the many drawbacks of aphakic spectacles, Ridley decided to see if a similar plastic could be used to make an artificial lens to replace the natural lens being removed in cataract surgery.

Ridley was the physician who courageously performed the first intraocular lens implant surgery in 1949 in London. It was a monumental event in the history of ophthalmology. However, both lens design and surgical techniques were crude by today's standards, so his results weren't always satis-factory. Like many visionaries, Ridley and his ideas were initially ridiculed and opposed by the medical establishment. Most doctors felt that it was too risky to insert objects permanently into the eye, and the idea of lens implantation was nearly abandoned.

Fortunately, research continued, and after nearly twenty years of experimentation with IOL designs by numerous surgeons in several countries, the modern IOL was developed. Today's IOLs bring no unwanted magnification and provide the most natural vision possible. IOLs are permanent, require no handling or care, and come in a wide range of powers.

Types of IOLs

Monofocal IOLs

The vast majority of implanted IOLs are *monofocal lenses*. The "mono" refers to the fact that the lens provides the best focus at a single location. For example, the lens may provide focus for seeing up close or far away, but not for both. Most patients prefer to have relatively good distance focus without glasses. This means that near objects will be very blurred

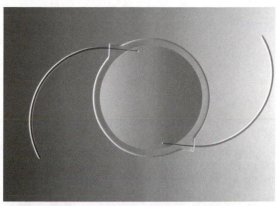

The monofocal IOL, shown above, is the standard IOL. Two flexible supports on each side act as tension-loaded springs that center the lens. IOL photos courtesy of Advanced Medical Optics.

without reading glasses. Accordingly, in order to see both up close and far away, an individual may choose from the same options of bifocals, trifocals, reading glasses, or contact lenses.

Multifocal IOLs

In 1997, the FDA approved the first *multifocal intraocular lens*, which provides focus for both distance and close work. Most of this lens is set for distance focus, but a portion is set for closer focus. The goal is to reduce one's dependence on eyeglasses by providing some ability to see close without them. Most patients with multifocal IOLs will still require

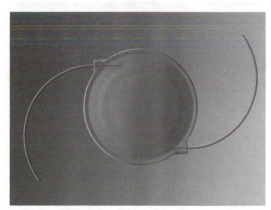

The multifocal IOL provides focus at both near and far distances.

glasses for some close tasks, depending upon factors such as lighting, the size and contrast of the print, or the task. Because they are associated with some slight optical tradeoffs, this type of IOL is generally chosen by a relatively small percentage of patients. More information on the multifocal IOL is provided in Chapter Eight.

Toric IOLs

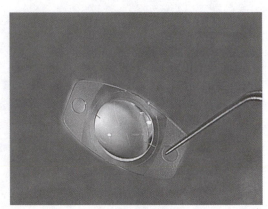

In 1998, the FDA approved the first IOL specifically designed to reduce high degrees of astigmatism. Called a *toric IOL*, it incorporates a special curvature (toric curve) into the IOL and can be implanted through a small incision. This design can reduce one's dependence on strong, astigmatism-correcting spectacles. However, since it is a monofocal IOL, patients still need glasses to read.

The toric IOL has a special curve and is used for patients with severe astigmatism.

Because severe astigmatism is not common, toric IOLs are used for a relatively small percentage of patients.

Accommodating IOLs

An *accommodating IOL* is designed to help one see objects both far away and near without eyeglasses. This artificial lens simulates the way the natural lens once moved as it changed our focus from far to close; you may recall, this process is called accommodation. The accommodating IOL acts on the same premise—it moves slightly back and forth along the axis of the eye in response to the movement of eye muscles.

The first model of the accommodating IOL was approved by the FDA in 2004 and tends to work best in those individuals who are hyperopic (farsighted.)

Unlike other IOLs for cataract surgery, the accommodating IOLs are not covered by medical insurance such as Medicare, and the cost is several thousand dollars. This limits their applicability for most cataract patients. Research continues on other special implant designs that could reduce one's dependence on reading glasses.

Secondary IOLs

Some patients may not have received an IOL at the time of their original cataract surgery many years ago. Even if the natural supportive lens capsule has been surgically removed, an IOL can still be implanted many years later. This type of IOL is called a *secondary IOL* implant because it is inserted during a second operation. Several different designs can be used for secondary IOLs, depending upon where, within the eye, the IOL can be best supported. Some IOLs are especially modified to allow them to be sewn into place. If you need a secondary IOL, your surgeon will determine which design is optimal based upon your eye's unique anatomy.

What Is an IOL Made of?

The early intraocular lenses were made of clear, rigid plastic, much like a hard contact lens. However, modern IOLs are made of either silicone or acrylic plastic and are foldable. Why is the ability to fold the IOL important? Folding the lens—or rolling or otherwise compressing it—allows it to be implanted through a much smaller incision. Foldable lenses are also associated with less frequent clouding of the posterior capsule, which is the portion of the capsular bag that supports the IOL. Although they are more expensive to manufacture, foldable lenses are now the preferred lens implant in developed countries.

Placement of the IOL

When the IOL is placed in front of the iris, it is called an *anterior chamber IOL*. If it is placed in the capsular bag behind the iris, it is referred to as a *posterior chamber IOL*. There is no difference in optical quality, vision, or comfort between the two types of IOLs. The anterior chamber IOL was preferred in the earlier period when cataract surgeons were limited to techniques that removed the entire lens. As surgical techniques evolved that allowed the capsular bag to be preserved for lens support, the posterior chamber IOL became the preferred design.

Commonly Asked Questions about IOLs

How long have IOLs been used?

The first IOLs in North America were used in the early 1970s; however, at first only a few surgeons used them. The use of IOLs became prevalent in the early 1980s, and today they are used by all surgeons in the developed world.

How long will the IOL last?

The IOL is permanent and, unlike an artificial joint or heart valve, there are no moving parts to wear out. Even artificial lenses implanted in children following congenital cataract surgery are expected to last a lifetime.

Can the IOL be removed and replaced?

Although it is rarely necessary, the IOL can be removed and replaced. The most common reason would be that the power is incorrect, despite all of the preliminary calculations. Another reason would be if the IOL shifted out of position inside the eye, a very rare event. Because the artificial lens is designed to be permanent, removing it is not a simple task.

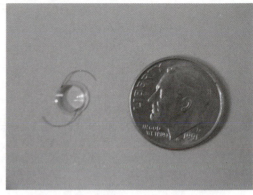

The photo above shows the relative size of a standard IOL, which measures about one-fourth inch across.
Photo by James McKinney.

Does the IOL replace the need for sunglasses?

Sunglasses provide two benefits. Their darker tint reduces the brightness of our surroundings by decreasing the amount of light that reaches the eye. The major health benefit is that they contain a transparent UV coating that blocks the ultraviolet rays of the sun. Ultraviolet rays are what cause sunburn and are present even on overcast days. Because of the potential for cumulative damage to the retina, it is advisable to block out ultraviolet light. All modern IOLs are permanently coated to provide this UV protection at all times. Since IOLs have no dark tinting, patients may still choose to wear sunglasses for comfort, just as they did before their cataract surgery.

Where are IOLs manufactured?

Although IOLs are manufactured in many industrialized countries, the IOLs commonly used in North America are produced in the United States. The quality control is very strict and of the highest standard to obtain FDA approval. In the non-indus-trialized world, inexpensive IOLs may be produced locally; these are not subject to the rigid standards of the FDA.

How is the IOL paid for?

In most surgical facilities, the IOL cost is either absorbed into a single flat fee for the operation, or it is part of a cost allowance determined by the insurer, such as Medicare. The hospital or surgery center purchases the IOL from the manufacturer, and the price is then incorporated into the surgical facility fee. Foldable IOLs are more expensive than the non-foldable lenses; multifocal IOLs and toric (astigmatic) IOLs are the most expensive. Surgical and facility fees for cataract surgery are usually set by the insurer or the local government. The patient generally pays the same fee regardless of the type of IOL used but may have to pay the additional costs for special IOLs.

5

Planning for Cataract Surgery

Being diagnosed with cataracts can produce feelings of anxiety. Understandably, anything that goes wrong with our eyes can feel scary. Fortunately, vision problems caused by cataracts are reversible. Today, cataract removal is one of the most successful surgeries done in North America, with several million procedures performed annually. The number is expected to grow as the population ages.

If you have cataracts that are causing vision problems, you and your ophthalmologist will need to decide when it's time to remove them. Once cataracts form, there are no medications, eyedrops, exercises, glasses, supplements, or herbs that can cause them to disappear. Cataracts must be removed through a surgical procedure, and a new, artificial lens—the intraocular implant—must be inserted to restore vision.

The good news is that, once removed, a cataract will never come back. And you're never too old to have cataract surgery because you're never too old to enjoy the benefits of better vision. Unfortunately, some people try to adapt to poorer vision, accepting it as a normal part of aging. However, they often do not realize how poor their vision has actually become. Nor do they realize how much their vision could be improved with cataract surgery.

When Should Cataracts Be Removed?

You should consider having cataract operation when its removal would noticeably improve your vision. Cataracts progress at surprisingly different rates. Some cataracts hardly seem to change for years, and others progress quickly. It is virtually impossible for your doctor to predict how quickly your cataract will progress. As cataracts inevitably worsen, the need for surgery becomes more obvious over time.

Your lifestyle and occupational needs should be central to your decision. For example, if your job or hobby requires excellent eyesight, you might elect to have surgery much earlier than someone who doesn't have the same vision requirements. You'll also want to consider the rate at which your vision is declining. Talk with your eye doctor about how your cataracts are affecting your vision and your life. Although your doctor cannot make the final decision for you, he or she can help you sort out the pros and cons.

Here are some questions you might ask your doctor:

- Would new eyeglasses improve my vision?
- Would I be able to pass a driving test right now?
- Is my cataract mild, medium, or advanced?
- Would the improvement from cataract surgery be subtle or obvious?
- Do I have any other problems besides cataracts that are reducing my vision?
- Does my eye's condition pose any special problems or risks for cataract surgery?
- What restrictions will I have following surgery?

- If I have surgery, how long will I be off work?
- If I currently need strong prescription glasses to see, what will my prescription be like following surgery?
- Is surgery covered by my insurance? If not, how much will it cost?

Having a cataract diagnosed doesn't mean you have to have it removed immediately. Most people have plenty of time to decide when to have cataract surgery. You and your doctor can decide when to have your cataracts removed based on how much the cataract is impairing your vision.

Who Performs Cataract Surgery?

General ophthalmologists perform cataract surgery. You'll want an ophthalmologist who is experienced. Good cataract surgeons are much like good golfers: they are trained well and have developed their skills through much practice. Based on years of experience, they are prepared for almost any situation and can perform well under pressure. As you'd expect, ophthalmologists who perform a greater number of cataract surgeries are more likely to have the most current and well-honed skills.

Finding the Right Cataract Surgeon

If your cataracts have been diagnosed and followed by an optometrist or an ophthalmologist who doesn't perform cataract surgery, you will need a referral to a cataract surgeon when you are ready for surgery. Your current eye doctor will usually be able to recommend a good cataract surgeon for you. After receiving the recommendation, ask your eye doctor if he or she has cared for others who have had their cataracts removed by that surgeon. You also can ask friends, family, coworkers, and other physicians for recommendations.

Check to see that your ophthalmologist is board-certified. This means he or she has passed a vigorous examination given by a board of peers. Take the time to learn about his or her credentials through the doctor's office brochure or web site.

When you meet with the surgeon, it is important that he or she makes you feel comfortable. You should be able to ask questions and have them answered in a manner that you understand. Becoming knowledgeable about cataracts, gaining confidence in your surgeon, and maintaining a positive attitude about your condition can help make your cataract surgery experience much easier.

Selecting Your Lens Implant Power

At some point prior to your surgery, your doctor will need to determine the power of the IOL that will replace the optical power once provided by your natural lens. IOLs are available in more than 65 different powers. The central viewing zone of the IOL, which provides the optical power, is called the *optic*. This is a clear, round disc measuring 6.0 mm in diameter (about ¼ inch). As with other types of lenses, the optical power of IOLs is measured in units called *diopters*.

Your surgeon will select a specific lens power for your IOL with the goal of achieving your target focal distance. With your input, the surgeon must decide approximately where (far, intermediate, or near focus) to target your uncorrected vision (without glasses) after IOL surgery. Your lifestyle, the vision of your other eye, and your prior eyeglass prescription are factors to consider.

If, for instance, it's especially important for you to be able to read up close without glasses, you may prefer to remain nearsighted after cataract surgery.

For others, a slight amount of myopia (nearsightedness) may represent a good compromise between having very blurred vision for either far distance or near distance without glasses. Some people elect to have one eye be focused for distance vision without glasses, and the other for a closer distance. This is called *monovision*. Not everyone, however, can comfortably adjust to this imbalance in focal distance.

Compounding the challenge of choosing a proper lens implant power is the fact that you cannot try out different powers of IOLs, as you can try out different lenses when getting eyeglasses or contact lenses. Since the IOL is placed inside the eyeball after the natural lens has been removed, there is no way to preview different IOL powers in advance.

The biggest advance in cataract surgery in the last decade has been the "small incision surgery," which requires no sutures.
—Dr. Howard Gimbel

Instead, your surgeon will use a computer program to help estimate an appropriate IOL power before surgery. The computer calculations are based on the dimensions of your eyeball. Performed in the doctor's office, these painless measurements determine the amount of corneal curvature, which correlates with the cornea's optical power, and the distance from the cornea to the retina. Since this distance cannot be determined with a ruler, ultrasound (medical sonar) or similar technology is used to measure this distance in tenths of a millimeter.

One of the recent advances in IOL power selection has been the development of a new method of measuring the retinal position called the IOL Master, approved by the FDA in 2000. This device uses a scanning diagnostic laser beam to measure the precise location of the retina to within one-hundredth of a millimeter. Like existing ultrasound technology, the IOL Master is safe, painless, and fast. Several studies have shown that the IOL Master provides the most accurate measurement.

Finally, it is important to remember that even with refinements in taking measurements for IOL power, determining target focus and selecting an appropriate lens implant power is an imperfect process. For example, another variable affecting the outcome is the IOL's position inside the eyeball, which the doctor must estimate prior to the surgery. Still, eyeglasses can always be prescribed to optimize your distance vision after cataract surgery.

> *Since cataracts become worse over time. Each person must decide not whether, but when to have surgery.*
> —Dr. David Chang

How a Cataract Is Removed

The preferred technique for cataract removal is called *extracapsular surgery.* There are two alternatives or techniques for doing this surgery: a small-incision method or a large-incision surgery. In both methods, the surgeon removes a small portion from the front of the capsule, the outer covering of the lens. As you may recall from the earlier discussion of eye anatomy, the capsule is a thin, transparent covering that encases the natural lens. During extracapsular surgery, the remaining capsular bag (outer covering of the lens) is left intact when the cloudy lens is removed. This provides a supporting sac-like structure to hold the artificial lens implant. Extracapsular surgery is a refinement of the surgical method of more than two decades ago, called *intracapsular surgery*, in which the entire lens and capsule were removed.

Small-Incision Surgery

The most common extra capsular surgical technique in North America is *small-incision surgery*. An estimated 95 percent of ophthalmologists use this technique. As the name implies, only a small incision, measuring approximately 3 millimeters (about 1/8 inch) is required.

Once the incision is made, the cataract is removed with an instrument called a *phacoemulsifier*. This instrument, originally designed in the 1970s, has been revolutionized by computer technology. Once inserted, the phacoemulsifier uses ultrasound waves, vibrating at 40,000 times per second, to break up the cloudy lens. This process is called *phacoemulsification*, or *phaco* for short. The pieces of lens are gently vacuumed out, and the new, foldable intraocular lens is inserted into the empty capsular bag, where it unfolds to its full size. Over a period of several weeks, the capsular bag contracts, essentially shrink-wrapping around the lens implant and holding it firmly in place.

Sutures are usually not required because the tiny incision is

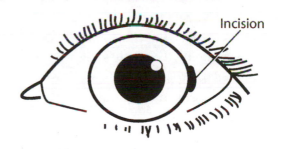

Small Incision

Incision

The newer small-incision surgery involves a tiny incision, about one-eighth inch. Outward pressure from fluid within the eye seals it. Usually, no sutures are required.

41

Advantages of Small-Incision Surgery

- Surgery can be performed more quickly

- Topical anesthesia can be used instead of local anesthesia

- Safer, if patient accidentally moves or coughs during surgery

- Permits the use of the newer, foldable IOLs

- No need for sutures

- Faster healing

- Generally no need to restrict exercise or physical activity

- Quicker recovery of sight

- New eyeglasses can be prescribed much sooner

- Less risk of the procedure creating or worsening astigmatism

- Less frequent need to change eyeglasses in the future

fashioned into a flap that closes on its own. Because the incision is so small, actions such as coughing, straining, or inadvertently rubbing the eye are not harmful. Accordingly, physical activities are not restricted after small-incision surgery.

Large-Incision Surgery

The large-incision method was the most popular procedure prior to the 1990s. In large-incision surgery, the solid central core of the cataract, called the *nucleus,* is removed intact rather than being broken apart by phaco. The nucleus makes up 90 percent of the volume of the lens, requiring a larger incision to remove it in one piece. The incision for this procedure is up to 12 millimeters long (one-half inch), compared to 1/8th of an inch for small incision surgery. Closing the large incision might require eight or nine sutures. Some doctors who are not experienced in small-incision surgery still use this method. Occasionally, a patient is a poor candidate for small-incision surgery; the cataract may be too dense to remove with ultrasound or the capsular bag may be too weak to allow phaco. These patients can have large-incision extracapsular cataract surgery and do well.

Since a large-incision procedure weakens the wall of the eye, a patient must limit physical activity for up to four weeks. Even bending over to tie a shoe can strain the incision as blood rushes to the head.

The large-incision procedure also causes greater changes in the

Large Incision

Large-incision cataract surgery requires an incision up to one-half inch. It is no longer the preferred method.

shape of the cornea, which can increase astigmatism. Overly tight sutures may cause excessive astigmatism that requires cutting the offending sutures after six weeks. For this reason, people might receive a temporary eyeglass prescription initially and a final eyeglass prescription several months later. To protect the eye from injury and to prevent rupturing the sutures by accidental rubbing, a patient wears a guard over the eye while sleeping.

6

Undergoing Cataract Surgery

Not so long ago, cataract surgery involved an overnight stay in the hospital. Today, cataract surgery is performed on an outpatient basis. The procedure is usually done in an outpatient surgery center or in the outpatient department of a hospital. Some cataract surgeons have surgical facilities adjoining their offices. Since they are surgical procedures, cataract operations should be performed in fully equipped operating rooms under antiseptic conditions to minimize the risk of infection.

Once you arrive at the surgery center, several steps will be taken to prepare you for your cataract removal. Although the surgery itself takes less than half an hour, because of the preoperative preparations and paperwork involved, you'll likely spend several hours at the surgery center.

Prior to Surgery

Using Eyedrop Medications

One or more days prior to surgery, you may be asked to use antibiotic eyedrops, and your eye doctor will instruct you in their use. The drops are intended to kill any bacteria that could cause an infection. Properly using prescribed eyedrop medications before and after surgery is important to the success of your cataract surgery. If you've never used eyedrops, it may take just bit of practice to get them into your eye—the natural reflex is to blink to avoid the drops. But it shouldn't take you long to learn how to use them properly.

The goal is to have the drop land anywhere on the exterior surface of the eyeball, then gently close your eye. Don't blink. The medication will spread across the eyeball's surface, and within a few minutes, will penetrate the cornea to reach the eye's interior.

It is important not to blink to much after putting in eyedrops. Blinking pumps the eyedrop medication from the eye surface toward the openings of the tear ducts. To reduce blinking, gently close the eye without squeezing the lids for at least a minute after putting in the drop.

> *Cataract surgery is not an unpleasant experience. Most patients experience no pain during the surgery.*
> —Dr. Howard Gimbel

The eyedrop will be effective if it lands on either the eyeball or in the pinkish inside surface on the lower eyelid. However, if the eyedrop lands on the eyelid skin or on the lashes, you'll have to try again.

Always wash your hands before using eyedrops. Eyedrop instillation is easiest if you either lie down or tilt your head back.

You need only one eyedrop of medication for one dose. Don't worry if you accidentally apply several drops; it won't harm the eye. If you think you missed your eye, it's okay to apply another drop. For more than one type of eyedrop medication, allow three or more minutes between each type of medication.

While you're first learning to use eyedrops, you may want to refrigerate your eyedrops. This makes it easier to tell whether the drop lands on the eyeball. Some people rely on a spouse or other family member to help them with eyedrops. Even if you have this

Inserting Eyedrops

1

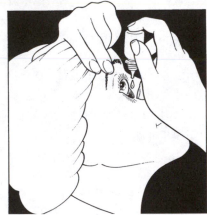

If you are right-handed, use the thumb and the first two fingers of your right hand to hold the inverted eyedrop bottle.

2

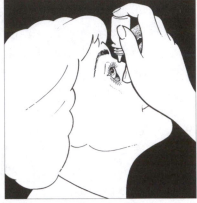

Hold the eyelid open by using your left index finger for the upper lid, and your right pinky finger for the lower lid.

3

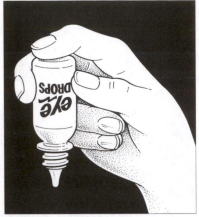

Hold the inverted bottle directly over your eye. Look at or slightly to the side of the bottle. Squeeze the bottle lightly with your fingertips to release one drop.

4

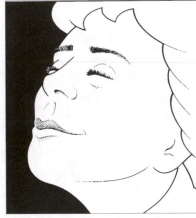

Once the eyedrop lands, keep the eyelids gently closed for 1-3 minutes.

46

option, it's better if you learn to do it for yourself in case your helper isn't available.

Other Medications

Continue taking your regular health medications, such as blood pressure medication, unless your surgeon tells you otherwise. Many ophthalmologists even allow their patients to continue taking aspirin and other blood thinners, because the risk of serious internal bleeding with small-incision cataract surgery and topical anesthesia is extremely low.

Food and Drink

Depending on the time of your scheduled surgery, your doctor may ask you not to eat or drink anything on the morning of your operation. If so, you might wish to have a snack before going to bed the night before so you don't feel too hungry. If you're diabetic and take insulin, your doctor may ask you to reduce or skip your morning dose before surgery.

> *Most patients are surprised at how easy it is to undergo cataract surgery. The procedure is quick and discomfort is usually minimal.*
>
> —Dr. David Chang

Before Leaving Home

- Make sure you have your insurance cards and related information. Some surgery centers may request that you complete a brief health questionnaire.
- Know who is going to drive you home. Because you'll be receiving mild sedation during surgery, this arrangement is necessary. If you don't have a family member or friend who can drive you home, ask your ophthalmologist's staff about possible alternatives.

- Wear loose, comfortable clothing.
- Do not apply makeup.
- Leave jewelry and valuables at home.
- If you take nitroglycerin pills or use inhalers for asthma or other breathing problems, take them along.

Preoperative Preparations

In the preoperative area, you'll be asked to change into a special, loose-fitting hospital gown. Depending on the facility, you'll be asked to sit in a chair or lie on a bed. If you have any problems lying flat, be sure to tell the nurse so the bed can be adjusted to make you comfortable. During this presurgery period, a friend or family member may usually keep you company.

A nurse will measure your vital signs, blood pressure, and heart rate. To help you relax, you'll probably be given a mild anti-anxiety medication. An intravenous (I.V.) line may be started in your arm or hand so that sedative medication can be administered during surgery as needed. The sedatives will probably not put you to sleep, but might make you drowsy and you may not remember parts of the procedure.

The nursing staff will administer eyedrop medications into the eye undergoing the procedure. Some surgery centers use a tiny, soft sponge called a *pledget* to administer eye medications. The nurse will gently place the pledget

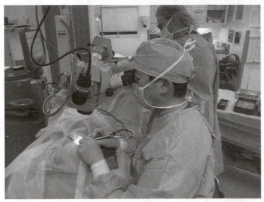

Eye surgeons use a microscope to perform cataract surgery.

underneath the eyelid in the corner where it won't bother you. One such medication will be dilating drops that are much stronger and take longer to work than those used in routine eye exams. Because of the strength of these eye drops, your pupil may still be dilated the next day.

Some people doze off during this time. Others bring a portable music player and headphones to pass the time.

Receiving Anesthesia

Cataract surgery is generally associated with minimal discomfort. Two types of anesthesia, both local, are commonly used for the procedure. Many doctors use topical anesthesia given as eyedrops. Other doctors use a regional anesthesia, which is administered by injection. The choice of anesthesia will depend on your surgeon's preference. Both types numb the eyeball well.

In years past, regional anesthesia, a longer-acting anesthesia delivered by injection, was the most commonly used anesthetic for cataract surgery. Nowadays, topical anesthesia is the preference of many surgeons. Topical anesthesia, however, can be used only with small-incision surgery.

Only in special cases would a doctor use general anesthesia, which puts the patient to sleep. For example, general anesthesia may be used for patients who can't cooperate, such as children or adults with dementia.

Regional Anesthesia

If you are having a regional anesthetic, your doctor will inject Novocain or a similar agent into your lower eyelid. This numbs the eyeball by anesthetizing the nerves leading to it. After the surgery, an eye patch must be worn until the anesthetic wears off. Why an eye patch? The longer-acting anesthetic injection temporarily weakens the muscles that control blinking, the eye's defense mechanism against drying and having something touch its surface. For this reason, the eye must be kept covered until the anesthetic agents wear off, which can take many hours. For most patients, the patch will be removed the following morning.

Topical Anesthesia

If you are having topical anesthesia, the doctor will administer anesthetic eyedrops. Patients usually require less sedation during surgery when they receive anesthesia in this way. Another one of the main advantages to topical anesthesia is that it avoids the potential side effects from the needle injection such as possible discomfort, bruising, swelling, or temporary drooping of the eyelids. And because the topical medication does not affect the surrounding muscles, no eye bandage is required at the end of the surgery.

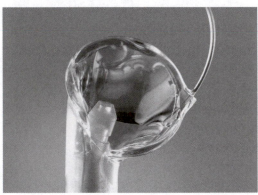

This foldable IOL is shown emerging from an injector used to insert the lens into the eye's capsular bag.
Courtesy of Advanced Medical Optics

Undergoing Small-Incision Cataract Removal

Before your procedure, the nurse will cleanse the skin around your eye and cover your eyelids with a sterile plastic drape. Once the surgeon begins the operation, he or she will use a device called a *speculum* to gently hold the eyelids open so you cannot blink. You will be able to see light but not the instruments being used. In fact, patients commonly report that they see a kaleidoscope of beautiful colors and radiating light patterns during their operation. Patients are also aware of a cool, wet sensation as eye drops are used to rinse and moisten the cornea throughout the surgery. Although few patients report discomfort, many say they feel pressure on their eyeball at times during the procedure.

With the help of a high-powered operating microscope, the surgeon performs cataract surgery inside the eye. The following steps are involved in a small-incision procedure:

- The small incision in the cornea is made using an ultrathin blade, often made from a diamond.
- A circular opening is made in the front of the lens capsule.
- The tip of the phacoemulsification instrument is inserted through the incision into the opened capsular bag.
- The cloudy lens is broken up by the phacoemulsifier. The pieces are gently suctioned out.
- The intraocular lens is folded and inserted through the incision. The artificial lens unfolds to its permanent shape.
- The incision is fashioned as a flap valve that closes on its own. No stitches are required.
- A special saline eyedrop solution is administered to reestablish proper intraocular pressure.

You'll be able to talk to the surgeon during the operation. For example, if you need to cough or sneeze, you can tell the doctor

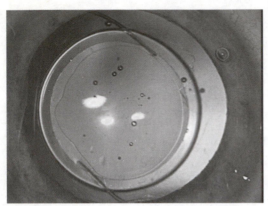

An IOL is shown here after implantation in an eyeball. The pupil has been dilated.
Courtesy of American Academy of Ophthalmology

Benefits of Cataract Surgery

- Improved eyesight

- Improved color vision and night vision

- Improved functional abilities for reading, driving, and occupational tasks

- For those with large preoperative refractive errors, a decrease in eyeglass prescription

- Less frequent need to change eyeglasses in the future

- A permanent end to the progressive worsening in vision caused by cataracts

so he or she can stop momentarily. Many patients remark about how quickly the actual surgical procedure is performed.

After Your Surgery

After the procedure, you'll be taken to a recovery room, where you'll rest briefly. The length of time needed to remain at the surgery center varies for each individual. Most patients are ready to be driven home within fifteen minutes.

Before you change into your street clothes and return home, a nurse will check your pulse and blood pressure once more and review the immediate postoperative instructions with you. Since the sedative often makes it hard to remember details, many doctors send you home with written instructions.

With small-incision surgery, you'll find you have few restrictions following surgery. If your surgeon has used topical anesthesia, you won't require an eye bandage. Because your eye was dilated during surgery, you will probably be more comfortable wearing sunglasses

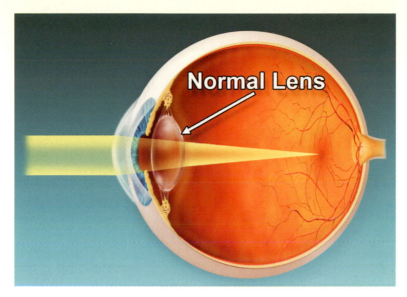

This illustration represents how light normally passes through the lens of the eye and focuses on the retina. Images are then sent to the brain for interpretation.

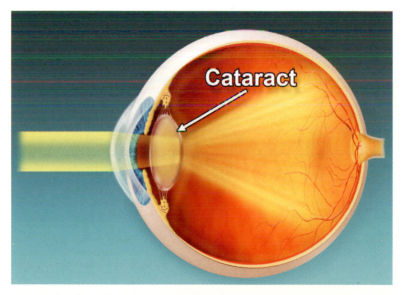

Here, the lens has become cloudy due to the formation of a cataract. As a result, light rays are scattered and cannot focus precisely on the retina.

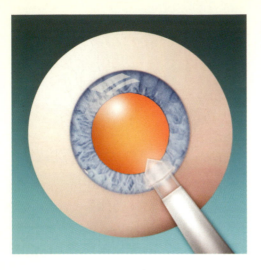

Small-Incision Cataract Surgery

1. First an incision, less than one-eighth inch, is made in the cornea.

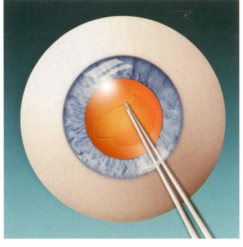

2. The surgeon creates an opening in the capsular bag, the thin membrane surrounding the lens. This membrane is only four-thousandths of a millimeter thick.

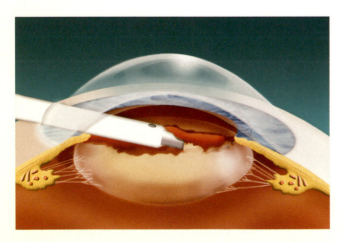

3. With the phacoemulsification technique, the surgeon uses an instrument shaped like a hollow needle. This side view shows how the ultrasound vibrations break the cataract into smaller pieces. The pieces are then suctioned from the eye with the same instrument.

4. The intraocular lens is folded and an "injector" is used to insert it into the capsular bag, where the lens unfolds. The foldable IOL makes it possible to keep the incision small.

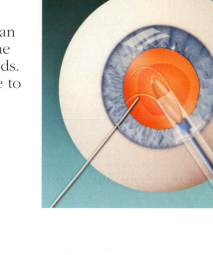

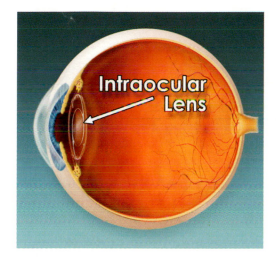

Intraocular Lens

5. This side view shows the implanted IOL in the capsular bag, which once held the natural lens.

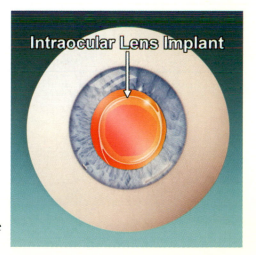

Intraocular Lens Implant

6. The frontal view of the implanted IOL demonstrates how the tiny "springs" on each side of the IOL keep it centered. Once the IOL has been placed, the surgery is complete. Sutures are usually not required. The incision self-seals like a one-way valve.

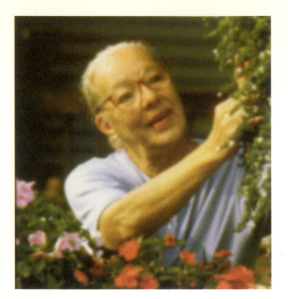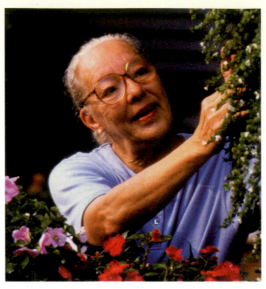

The photos above present how a cataract can cause color distortion. The photo with the yellow cast on the left was before cataract surgery. The photo on the right represents the vision improvement after surgery. *Courtesy of American Academy of*

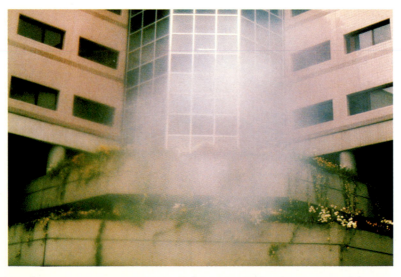

Another common symptom of cataracts is glare caused by incoming light. This photo represents glare caused by a cataract. *Courtesy of American Academy of Ophthalmology*

outdoors. The pupil will often remain dilated for more than 24 hours.

In most cases, you will have a follow-up visit with your surgeon the next day. During the follow-up visit, any sedative will have worn off, and you will likely feel more clear-headed. This will be a better time to ask questions about any long-term concerns you have.

Potential Risks

For most people, the chance of successful cataract surgery is greater than 98 percent. As with any operation, complications are possible, but severe problems that can cause permanent vision loss are rare. For example, the chance of major internal bleeding is less than one in 1,000. The risk of infection is less than one in 1,000.

Rare but unpredictable complications can occur with regional (local injection) or general anesthesia. Other uncommon, but possible complications include:

- Prolonged elevation of intraocular pressure
- Persistent internal eye inflammation called *iritis*
- Macular edema caused by microscopic amounts of fluid pooling in the center of the retina
- Corneal clouding caused by the depletion of cells which keep the cornea clear
- Problems with the retina, such as retinal detachment

Complications such as elevated pressure, iritis, and macular edema are treatable with eyedrop medications. Permanent corneal clouding and retinal detachment are rare unless you are prone to these two condition. If they should occur, both are treated with surgery. If you are concerned about complications, discuss them with your eye surgeon.

Call your ophthalmologist immediately if you have any of the following symptoms after surgery:

- Severe pain not relieved by nonprescription pain medication
- Sudden loss of vision
- Injury to the eye
- Stringy yellow or green discharge from the eye

Treatment for Cataracts in Both Eyes

If you have cataracts in both eyes, your cataract surgery will be performed on one eye at a time on different days. This is the standard of care for cataract removal. Since you will likely have temporary blurred vision from cataract surgery, your doctor wants to avoid your having blurred vision in both eyes during the healing process. Also, waiting to operate on the second eye lets the surgeon assess the intraocular lens power chosen for the first procedure.

How soon can you have surgery on the second eye? This will depend on how quickly your first eye recovers. Typically, cataract removal on the second eye takes place a few weeks after the first operation. Under rare circumstances, however, it may be possible for a person to have both operations within the same week. For example, if someone travels from out of town for the surgery, the second procedure might be scheduled within the week to accommodate the patient.

7

Recovering from Surgery

Your cataract surgery is over. You are the recipient of a new artificial lens, one of the amazing accomplishments of modern medicine! Your cataract will never come back, and your new intraocular lens will never cloud.

If you are like the majority of individuals, you probably found that the entire cataract surgery experience was quicker and much easier than you expected. Over the next few days, your eyeball will be healing.

Returning to See Your Doctor

You'll probably have an appointment to see your eye surgeon at his or her office the morning after your operation. This visit allows the doctor to check the condition of your eye and its intraocular pressure. The doctor will also explain how often and how long you need to use postsurgical eyedrop medications. This is also a good opportunity for you to ask any questions you might have.

Your doctor will conduct only a very limited vision test during this first visit after surgery. Naturally, you're curious about the results of your cataract surgery. Many people needlessly worry because they aren't seeing well immediately after surgery. Blurred vision and other temporary postsurgical effects are common during recovery. They neither predict nor correlate with how well you'll see after your eye has healed.

Common Symptoms after Surgery

Immediately following your cataract surgery, you may experience a number of the following symptoms, which are normal and will disappear over time:

- Blurred and fluctuating vision
- Sensitivity to bright light
- Dilated pupil for one or two days
- Watering eyes
- Scratchy, sandy feeling
- Eye redness
- Stinging from eyedrops
- Halos around lights at night
- Floaters

If you find you are sensitive to light, sunglasses may make you feel more comfortable. However, since your new, artificial lens blocks out ultraviolet light, it is not necessary to wear sunglasses for UV protection.

Causes of Temporary Blurred Vision

At first, your vision will probably be quite blurred. If you had large-incision cataract surgery, your blurry vision might persist for several weeks. However, if you had small-incision cataract surgery and you're like most people, you should notice your vision improving within a few days after your surgery. Keep in mind that these side effects are temporary. There are several reasons for the temporarily blurred vison.

Dilation of the Pupil

Immediately after your surgery, your pupil will still be dilated. As mentioned previously, the dilating drops used during surgery are stronger than the dilating drops used during eye exams. The effects of these drops may linger for more than 24 hours, and may cause you to see an assortment of reflections and halos.

Patients often describe seeing a "curved line of reflected light" from light sources at night. This is similar to a halo effect and may be particularly noticeable if your pupil tends to dilate very well in the dark. This reflected light effect occurs as light coming from the side enters the dilated pupil. When the light enters at just the right angle, it glances off the edge or surface of the intraocular lens and you see a momentary reflection.

> *The small incisions we use today in cataract surgery help patients heal much more quickly.*
> —Dr. Howard Gimbel

If you experience this side effect, be assured that it's normal and is a result of the IOL's design. Although it may be distracting at first, you'll notice these reflections less and less over time. Also, after several months, the remaining capsule holding the IOL tends to cloud slightly around the implant's edge, which acts to significantly reduce these reflections.

Misting of the Cornea

Misting in the cornea is caused by microscopic swelling, which is a normal response to surgery. This misting, which may last for several days, creates temporary blurring. This reaction

57

varies greatly among individuals. It will usually clear up during the first week.

Microscopic Movement of the IOL

After cataract surgery, some people notice a shimmering effect when they move their eyes. For example, at night when they look at car headlights or street lights, they might see what appears to be a slight movement of the lighted object. This occurs as a result of a slight movement of the IOL. As you recall, during surgery, the IOL is placed inside the empty capsular bag. During the first few weeks, the bag will contract and tighten around the artificial lens like a shrink-wrap. Until this happens, some slight jiggling movement of the IOL is normal. As a result of these slight movements, the eye's focus can vary during the first several days following surgery.

Wrinkle in the Capsular Bag

You may notice starburst reflections at night as a result of a tiny wrinkle in the back portion of the capsular bag that holds your IOL. As the capsular bag starts to shrink and contract around the implanted IOL, this light-scattering wrinkle will smooth out and disappear.

Recovery after Surgery

After surgery, your doctor will have given you thorough instructions for caring for your eye during the healing phase. Whether your doctor restricts your activities depends on the type of surgery you had—large- or small-incision.

After Small-Incision Surgery

It is more likely that you had small-incision cataract surgery. If so, you will have virtually no restrictions because the tiny incision does not weaken the wall of the eyeball. You can resume your everyday activities right away. You can also resume physical exercise such as golfing, jogging, or aerobics as soon as you wish. You don't have to worry about injury to your eye when you bend, stoop, lift, cough or strain. You can read, use your computer, or watch television as much as you want. Soap and water won't harm your eye, so you don't have to worry about showering, washing your face or hair or wearing makeup. You don't have to change your diet or alter your sleeping position. You can drive and return to work whenever you feel ready.

After Large-Incision Surgery

If you had the less common large-incision surgery, you'll have restrictions in movement and physical activity. You will need to avoid heavy lifting, bending, and straining for several weeks following surgery. Such activities increase blood flow to the head, which exerts external pressure against the eyeball and the incision.

You'll need to wear an eye patch immediately after surgery, and a protective eye shield at night for a few weeks. Your doctor may ask you to avoid getting water in the eye at first. Such guidelines will vary among doctors.

Using Eyedrops after Surgery

After your surgery, you will have been given a schedule for using eyedrops. Anti-inflammatory eyedrops will help decrease discomfort and light sensitivity and will speed healing. Antibiotic drops will prevent infection. These postsurgery medications are usually continued for several weeks, and your doctor will give you instructions on when to taper or eliminate their use. Note that it is common for the drops to cause some stinging, especially the first day or two.

If you wish, you can also take aspirin, Tylenol, or other over-the-counter pain relievers to help with any postoperative aching that isn't relieved by eyedrops or by taking a nap. In most cases, your eye will feel much better by the next morning.

Using Multiple Drops

You will likely be using several different kinds of eyedrop medications. You can administer them in any order–just make sure you allow three or more minutes between each medication. This way, the second drop won't rinse away the first one before it has had time to be absorbed.

Occasionally, when they finally stop using the postsurgery eyedrops, some people notice some scratchiness or mild irritation. This suggests a tendency toward "dry eye," a common and harmless condition that's much like dry mouth or dry skin. If you have this symptom, using over-the-counter lubricant drops called artificial tears can help to reduce the irritation. You can use artificial tears anytime, but most people wait until they have finished their postoperative eye medications before starting or resuming these over-the-counter eyedrops.

Don't Compare Your Recovery to Others'

Don't worry if your postsurgery experience, including restrictions on activities following surgery, is different from that of others you know who have undergone cataract surgery. They may have undergone a different surgical technique. For example, if a friend cautions you about bending over or lifting objects, the chances are that he or she had cataract surgery with a large incision. Comparing experiences can lead to considerable confusion. Following your surgeon's aftercare instructions, rather than the advice of friends and family, is your best bet.

Also, don't be concerned if your cataract surgery recovery rate is different from someone else's. Everyone heals at a different rate. Your recovery rate is normal for you. Some people even find differences in how they recovered from cataract surgery in each eye.

Wearing Your Eyeglasses after Surgery

Right after your cataract surgery, if your distance vision without glasses is good, you'll probably find you can't read well without glasses. While you wait for your new glasses, you might be able to wear an old pair of glasses for reading. Or, you may find that wearing over-the-counter reading glasses works. These inexpensive reading glasses are sold in most drug, grocery, stationery, and craft stores. They come in multiple standard powers ranging from +1.00 to +3.00 and are available in half or full spectacle frames.

If you want to try these standard over-the-counter reading glasses, but you're unsure what power to buy, simply try them on in the store to see which strength works best for you. Although these reading glasses won't work that well if your two eyes have different prescriptions, and they won't correct astigmatism, many people find that they provide a functional and inexpensive option until new reading glasses can be prescribed.

When Will New Eyeglasses Be Prescribed?

After cataract surgery, your eyeglass prescription will change. After small-incision surgery, your prescription will stabilize much faster than after large-incision surgery. You can usually have your new glasses prescribed within several weeks of surgery. If you order them too soon, you may need to have them revised. If you're having cataracts removed from both eyes, it's generally a good idea to wait until after the second operation to change your eyeglass prescription. You won't, of course, be able to fully evaluate your true distance and near vision capabilities until you have your new eyeglasses. As we discussed in the previous chapter, it may take several months for the eye to stabilize; then you can receive the best prescription for glasses.

Commonly Asked Questions about Recovery

When can I drive again?

There is no standard answer. Patients must decide for themselves at what point they see well enough to resume driving. Many patients are comfortable driving to their first postoperative visit on the morning after surgery. This is because surgery was performed on their worst eye, leaving the better eye unaffected. Obviously, if you feel your vision is not adequate, then you shouldn't drive.

How soon can I take the eye test for my driver's license?

Although some patients will be able to pass the eye test without glasses, it is best to wait until the final postoperative refraction and vision test is administered several weeks following surgery. This way, if new corrective lenses are prescribed, you will have them available for taking the test. Understanding this, your local Department of Motor Vehicles will usually grant an extension.

If I have cataract surgery and an IOL is inserted, can I wear contacts?

Yes. In fact, if you want to use the strategy of monovision (one eye set for far focus, and one eye set for near focus) to avoid glasses, it is far better to accomplish this with contact lenses. This way, the different focal points can be more precisely adjusted, and this state of differing vision is reversible, in case it later becomes a disadvantage.

How soon can I wear contacts after surgery?

Your previous contact lens will now have the wrong prescription. By the time a new lens is prescribed and fit, it will usually be at least one month after surgery and by then, you may wear them.

I don't like bifocals. Do I have to have them in my new eyeglasses?

As they are for everyone over the age of 45, bifocals are simply an alternative to wearing separate glasses for distance and reading. People who see well in the distance without glasses sometimes still prefer bifocals so that they don't have to take their reading glasses on and off.

Is there any way to tell me exactly what my vision will be without glasses after cataract surgery?

Unfortunately, because of the cataract's presence, it is impossible to demonstrate this to you in advance. Understandably, many patients are curious as to how well they will be able to see without glasses after surgery. This is difficult to describe because with IOL surgery, your surgeon cannot precisely control or achieve the exact focal distance for the eye that you might request. For instance, one patient might want the targeted focus to be far distance without glasses. Another patient might want their eye to be focused slightly closer without glasses. However, these are only targets. This also makes it particularly difficult to decide on certain options such as a multifocal IOL, because you cannot preview and compare both the advantages and disadvantages.

What Is a Secondary Membrane?

Several months or even years after cataract surgery, a small percentage of people, between 5 and 10 percent, will develop what is called a *secondary membrane*. This refers to a clouding of the back of the lens capsule. This membrane is also sometimes referred to as a "secondary cataract" or an "after cataract;" however, these terms are misleading since cataracts never recur once the natural lens has been removed.

Let's take a closer look at how these secondary membranes occur. Remember that a transparent capsule originally surrounded the natural lens. In cataract surgery, the front of this capsule is removed to allow for removal of the cloudy lens. The IOL is implanted into the empty capsule, which will then support and "shrinkwrap" around the artificial lens. The back of the capsular

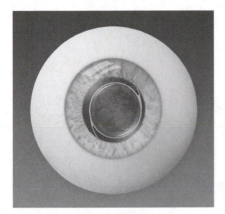

An eye with a secondary membrane. Notice the hazy capsule visible behind the lens.

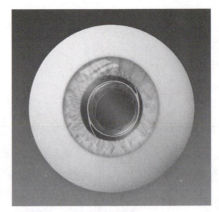

After a YAG procedure, the central haze is gone. The procedure is painless and takes only a few minutes in the doctor's office.

sac—called the posterior capsule—is left intact. So, after cataract surgery, we are looking through both the new artificial lens and the back of the original capsule.

Over time, in some eyes a layer of cloudy cells can gradually grow across the posterior capsule, much like dust gathering on a window. As a result, light cannot be focused clearly through this membrane, and the individual has a gradual progressive decline in vision, much like that caused by the original cataract. The most common symptoms are blurred or hazy vision; one may also experience glare.

A secondary membrane typically occurs one to three years after cataract surgery. Such a membrane is more likely to occur in younger patients, under sixty, who have had subcapsular cataracts, the ones that typically form along the back of the lens.

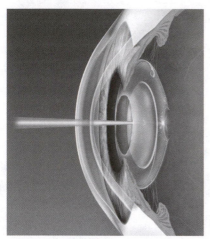

Months or years later, if a secondary "cataract" or membrane forms, a YAG laser procedure clears away the hazy layer of cells at the back capsule.

Fortunately, this condition is not a complication and it is not serious.

Treating a Secondary Membrane

If you develop a secondary membrane, which sufficiently blurs your vision, it is easily treated. A painless laser procedure, known as a *YAG capsulotomy*, and is performed in a matter of minutes in a doctor's office or clinic. YAG is short for Nd.YAG and refers to *neodymium yttrium aluminum garnet*, crystals that are the active medium in the laser used. The term capsulotomy means that a hole is made in the capsule.

Because of the small size of our pupils, we only look through the center of the IOLs and the posterior capsule. Therefore, it is not necessary to remove the entire clouded capsular bag in order to restore clear vision. Instead, a laser is used to make a small hole or "window" in the center of the posterior capsule to allow for a clear view. This permanent hole is about one-eighth inch in diameter and will not close later. The rest of the capsule remains intact to support the IOL just as securely as before.

Historically, a special knife or instrument would have been inserted through a surgical incision in the eye wall to create an opening. Since the mid-1980's however, the use of the YAG laser has eliminated the need for a surgical incision.

Undergoing a YAG Capsulotomy

For a YAG laser treatment, you will be seated at an eye microscope similar to that used for a routine eye exam. Anesthetic drops are all that will be needed to numb your eye.

A special focusing lens will be placed on your eye to control eye movements and to prevent the lids from closing. Because the amount of laser energy is so small, there is no danger to your other eye or other parts of your body. Although you should not feel any pain, you will notice a clicking sound as the laser is administered. This series of multiple clicks represents the many tiny applications used to create a small opening in the cloudy capsule. Each microscopic nick will result in a progressively larger opening until the optimal size is attained.

Following the treatment, your eye may be temporarily blurred for a few hours. You may also notice new temporary floaters. Your eye may be slightly irritated later in the day. Pain is uncommon and a bandage is not necessary. You may notice improvement in your vision later on that same day, or by the next morning. The laser treatment does not change your eyeglass prescription. The procedure will never have to be repeated because the optical hole in the capsule will always remain open.

Does a YAG Procedure Carry Risks?

Fortunately, risks for this procedure are minimal. In fact, the laser procedure avoids risks associated with actual surgery, such as bleeding or infection. Rarely, in predisposed eyes, changes in the eye fluid pressure and in the retina can occur after a laser procedure. You may notice floaters immediately following the laser treatment. These are microscopic particles from the capsule and will disappear. They are different from the permanent floaters in the vitreous gel that most patients develop as a result of aging.

8

Reducing Dependence on Eyeglasses

Some people mistakenly believe that having cataract surgery will enable them to see perfectly without glasses. Having the eye's natural cataract-clouded lens removed and replaced with a clear artificial lens can certainly improve your vision. However, the conventional artificial lens is a single, fixed-focus lens. It cannot provide distance focus one moment and near focus the next as the eye's natural lens does in a young person. So even after cataract surgery, prescription lenses will be needed to optimize and shift the focus of your eye. Still, there are options that may reduce your dependence on eyeglasses or contacts after cataract surgery.

Multifocal IOLs

One option which will reduce the need for glasses or contacts is the multifocal IOL; however, this decision should be made carefully. As mentioned in an earlier chapter, multifocal IOLs provide both near and far focus, so you will have some ability to see close without glasses. The near focus is best if both eyes have a multifocal IOL implant. However, because most of the lens optic is used for distance, most people with multifocal IOLs still find it easier to read with glasses, especially when reading small print or in low light or for long periods of time. Although the multifocal

IOL won't eliminate reading glasses, it may provide the convenience of reading many things without them.

Is a Multifocal IOL Right for You?

Although the multifocal IOL can reduce your dependence on eyeglasses, there are some trade-offs. The different focal zones of the lens optic create the appearance of halos around lights at night. If, for example, you look at a streetlight in the distance at night through a multifocal IOL, the streetlight would appear in sharp focus through the IOL's central distance zone. The peripheral near-focusing portion of the IOL, however, would make the streetlight appear blurry. This creates a slight ghost image or halo around the edge of the light. The halo effect isn't a problem during the daytime, but as the pupils normally dilate with less light at night, the ghost images become more evident. If you have extremely large pupils, the halo effect at night is increased.

> *Many patients don't understand that after cataract surgery they will still need eyeglasses for certain tasks.*
> —Dr. David Chang

Seeing halos is a distraction that doesn't really interfere with vision. Over time, most people's brains adapt to the images, and the halos become less noticeable and bothersome. People who have multifocal IOLs in both eyes have an easier time adjusting to the halos. However, not everyone can adapt. The multifocal design doesn't work well if one has significant astigmatism or other problems involving the cornea, macula, or optic nerve. If the pupil is too small, the patient cannot adequately see through the peripheral reading zone. Why would the pupil size matter? The multifocal IOL has a round optic. The central most region is set for distance focus. The peripheral areas are set for closer focus. When the pupil is small, the patient is viewing through only the center, or distance-focusing portion of the IOL. The pupil must be wide enough for light to pass through the more peripheral, near-focusing regions for the patient to see up close without glasses.

If the pupil is too large, the patient will experience more glare and halos at night. Some patients find that the halos create difficulty with night driving. Unfortunately, the doctor cannot tell in advance how someone will be affected by these symptoms.

Finally, the individual patient's lifestyle and activities should be considered. Whether a multifocal lens is right for you is something you and your eye doctor should decide together. Remember that both multifocal and standard monofocal IOLs will provide excellent vision following cataract surgery. If your eye doctor believes you're a good candidate for the multifocal IOL, and you want to reduce your dependence on eyeglasses, this lens may be an option for you. However, in many surgical practices, the multifocal IOL is implanted in fewer than 5 percent of patients.

Research continues on other multifocal IOL designs; so-called "accommodating" IOL designs are being tested as well. However, it will take a number of years to fully understand the long-term results.

Astigmatic Keratotomy

Another option for reducing the need for eyeglasses is a surgical procedure called *astigmatic keratotomy*. Astigmatism is a refractive error caused by a cornea that's shaped more like the side of a football, rather than the side of a perfectly round basketball. If you have significant astigmatism, details such as print or street signs appear blurred without glasses. The more astigmatism you have, the more blurred your uncorrected vision will be and the more dependent you'll be on eyeglasses or contact lenses.

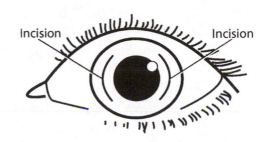

For an astigmatic keratotomy, a surgeon makes two small incisions on the cornea, making it more spherical like a basketball.

To perform astigmatic keratotomy, a surgeon uses special surgical blades made from diamonds to make precise incisions in the oblong cornea, allowing the cornea to become more round when it heals. By varying the length, depth, and locations of the incisions, the ophthalmologist can control how much change is made in the cornea's shape and curvature. The main risk with astigmatic keratotomy comes from improper incision depth, but this risk can be virtually eliminated if the surgeon uses specially designed "guarded" blades.

Although astigmatic keratotomy usually won't eliminate astigmatism completely, it can significantly reduce the blur and help you see more clearly without eyeglasses. It can also reduce how much correction must be used in your eyeglasses. Interestingly, this procedure is more effective the older you are.

Astigmatic keratotomy is a totally separate procedure from cataract removal. However, because the small incisions for astigmatic keratotomy are made in the cornea's external surface and don't weaken the eye in any way, they can be done at the same time as cataract surgery. It's fairly common to have both procedures done simultaneously, and having them done together does not prolong recovery time.

Astigmatic keratotomy is worth considering if your ophthalmologist thinks you are a candidate, and you are interested in enhancing your ability to see without glasses. Note that astigmatic keratotomy is an elective procedure and is usually not covered by health insurance. This procedure is more popular than the toric IOLs, also used to treat astigmatism.

Toric IOLs

Unlike eyeglasses, standard IOLs do not correct astigmatism. However, astigmatism-correcting intraocular lenses are now available. Called toric IOLs, these lenses can reduce the need for glasses or contacts.

How do these lenses work? Because astigmatism is caused by two different curvatures to the oblong cornea, some of the light is focused in front and some behind the retina. To correct this blur, the toric IOL must accomplish two things: First, the corrective lens must be approximately as oblong as the cornea. Second, the oblong axes of the cornea and of the corrective lens must be exactly aligned. Only then will the corrective lens match and compensate for the oblong cornea, to produce a sharp focus on the retina. If the corrective lens is misaligned or moves out of alignment, the focus remains blurred.

Like other posterior chamber IOLs, the toric IOL is permanently implanted into the capsular bag. It has a different shape, however, than that of standard IOLs. Unlike conventional posterior chamber IOLs, the toric IOL has four rounded corners.

Once the round capsular bag shrink-wraps the IOL during the first week following surgery, the corners prevent it from rotating.

However, during the first few days after surgery, the capsular bag still is loose, and it is possible for the toric IOL to rotate out of optimal alignment. If this happens, a tiny instrument can be inserted into the eye to rotate the lens back into proper and permanent alignment. Although this may require a trip back into the operating room, the procedure is quite minor. Fortunately, this happens infrequently.

As with astigmatic keratotomy, the toric IOL will usually not correct all of the astigmatism, especially if it is severe. Although it is difficult to eliminate astigmatism completely, any reduction will improve one's ability to see without glasses. Eyeglasses can correct whatever astigmatism remains. Your ophthalmologist will discuss whether either of these astigmatism-reducing options is appropriate for you. The toric design is usually reserved for severe astigmatism. In most surgical practices, it is used in less than 5 percent of cases.

Should I Wait for Better IOLs?

IOLs will certainly continue to evolve. You may wonder whether you should wait for the next new IOL design. Unfortunately, it might be a long wait. Even though research continues, product development and FDA approval of a new IOL design can take up to ten years. It takes so long, in part, because the safety of new medical devices like IOLs must be tested over many years. Future improvements in IOL technology should be of relatively modest impact.

You can enjoy the benefits of current IOL designs that have evolved over the past two decades and have a proven track record from being implanted in millions of eyes annually. Rest assured that all the IOLs used in North America have passed rigorous, long-term testing for optical quality, safety, and performance. Current IOL manufacturing in the United States is done under strict quality controls and meets the highest possible industry standards. If your vision is altered by cataracts, the immediate benefits of surgery far outweigh any minor refinements in IOLs that may appear in the future

Of course, with several choices now available in IOLs, you may be confused about which one to choose. Your eye surgeon can help. Tell your doctor about your preference for near or distance focus without glasses. Your surgeon will take your preferences into account, as well as your individual risk factors and the health of other structures inside your eye, and select the best IOL for you.

Secondary IOLs

Perhaps you had cataract surgery before IOLs were available and are wondering whether you can still have an IOL implanted now. The answer is yes, in most cases, you can. Such an implant is called a *secondary IOL*, and it can reduce the need for special glasses or contacts.

A number of people have undergone cataract surgery without receiving an IOL. Maybe someone had the operation years ago before IOLs were the standard. Or perhaps there were complications that made implanting an IOL inadvisable at the time. In some special cases, the natural lens was removed during retinal surgery with the idea of implanting an IOL at a later time. Whatever the reason, most people can have a second operation to implant an artificial lens.

An eye without a lens after cataract surgery is called *aphakic.* In order to see, most aphakic patients wear a special post-cataract contact lens. (In rare cases where both eyes are aphakic and the person cannot wear contacts, thick cataract glasses may be used, but they are a poor solution.) Although aphakic contacts can be inconvenient, they work well for many people and provide the same quality of vision possible with an IOL. Besides the inconvenience of having to remove them daily, the biggest problem with aphakic contacts is that the person is functionally blind without them.

A person who has been successfully wearing aphakic contact lenses may eventually elect to have a secondary IOL implanted for a number of reasons. As eyesight worsens with age or manual dexterity decreases with conditions like arthritis, handling the contacts may become more difficult. Dry eyes or corneal problems may cause irritation and reduce the time the contact lens can be worn each day. Contacts can also be lost or torn, which is both inconvenient and expensive.

Most aphakic patients can have a secondary IOL implanted at any time. This second operation carries slight risks, such as inflammation and bleeding; the risk varies depending on the condition of the eye after the first surgery. However, if the person has otherwise healthy eyes, the success rate for secondary IOL surgery is greater than 95 percent.

The type of IOL that can be used for a secondary IOL implantation depends on the anatomy of your eye after the original surgery. Your eye surgeon will determine the right IOL for you at the time of surgery. If enough of the lens capsule remains, it may support a posterior chamber IOL. If not, an anterior chamber IOL can be positioned in front of the iris. For some people, prior injuries or surgical complications have resulted in internal iris scarring or the removal of iris tissue that makes it impossible to support an anterior chamber IOL. Even in this case, posterior chamber IOLs can be permanently sutured into place.

LASIK Surgery

If you have had cataract surgery, you may be wondering if you can further improve your ability to see without glasses by having refractive surgery, such as LASIK. The answer is yes, you can have LASIK after cataract surgery, but the practice is not common. Before explaining why it is rarely done, let's first examine what LASIK does.

LASIK, which stands for *laser in situ keratomileusis*, is used to treat nearsightedness, farsightedness, and astigmatism. This popular procedure, approved by the Food and Drug Administration in 1999, reshapes the cornea of the eyeball with a computer-driven laser. To perform a LASIK procedure, an eye surgeon first passes an instrument with a blade across the cornea, making a flap in the outer portion of the cornea. The doctor then pulls back the flap and reshapes the cornea with a laser, which vaporizes tissue without causing heat damage. The computer-controlled laser is so sensitive it can remove the equivalent of one two-thousandth of a human hair in four billionths of a second. Once the cornea is reshaped, the thin flap is closed. The cornea heals without sutures.

So, why is LASIK not generally chosen after cataract surgery? Keep in mind that once you have an artificial lens—the IOL—you also cannot focus at different distances like you could with a natural lens before the age of 40. Just as with anyone else past his or her forties, patients who see reasonably well in the distance without glasses must wear reading glasses to bring the focus closer.

Now let's say that after IOL surgery, you end up slightly myopic (nearsighted). Although your distance vision won't be perfect without glasses, this isn't really a bad result. Having some myopia will probably allow you to see a number of things up close without glasses as long as they aren't too small. Having LASIK could further improve your ability to see far away or drive without glasses. However, you would then lose the partial ability to see some near objects without glasses. In most patients with IOLs, LASIK would accomplish better vision (without glasses) at one distance, at the expense of worse vision (without glasses) at another distance. This tradeoff wouldn't justify more surgery. Only if one's vision is far off from the intended refractive target would LASIK generally be worth considering.

Still, if you should wish to consider LASIK after cataract surgery, you would need to wait for several months before having the procedure. It is important for the eye to stabilize after the cataract surgery before having another surgical procedure. Because LASIK is intended to reduce one's dependence on glasses, most medical insurance providers, such as Medicare, will not cover the cost.

9

Special Conditions & Cataract Surgery

If you have health problems such as diabetes or other eye conditions such as glaucoma, high myopia, or macular degeneration, you may be concerned your condition will make you a poor candidate for surgery. It is of key importance to realize that if you have vision loss created by another eye condition, cataract surgery may not bring much vision improvement. On the other hand, advances in technology and the skill of your surgeon may allow you to reap the benefits of cataract surgery. Each situation must be evaluated on an individual basis. Your doctor will consult with you about the proper timing of surgery and how other eye or health conditions may influence the outcome of cataract surgery.

Diabetes

If you have diabetes, you already know that it is a medical condition that results in abnormally high levels of blood sugar. It is estimated that 17 million Americans, or 6 percent of the population, have diabetes. Diabetics are 60 percent more likely to develop cataracts and tend to develop them at an earlier age than they otherwise might.

Checking for Retinopathy

If you have diabetes and you have a cataract, your ophthalmologist will do a careful preoperative evaluation of your eye. The doctor will be checking for a condition known as diabetic retinopathy, which refers to cumulative damage to small blood vessels in the retina caused by elevated blood sugar levels. Nowadays, with proper medication and prompt eye treatment, most diabetics will not lose their vision to retinopathy.

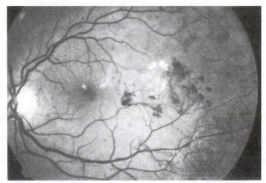

This patient has diabetic retinopathy. The dark spots are abnormal blood vessel formations and small hemorrhages.

If you do not have diabetic retinopathy, you should still expect an excellent outcome from cataract surgery. Diabetics about to undergo operations elsewhere in the body are often told that they may not heal as well as nondiabetics. Fortunately, this is not the case with small-incision cataract surgery; the incision is so small that healing is rapid.

Determining the Severity of Retinopathy

If you have diabetic retinopathy, the prognosis for cataract surgery depends on the severity of the condition. There are two forms of retinopathy, nonproliferative and proliferative. In the most common form, *nonproliferative diabetic retinopathy*, the capillaries in the retina become leaky and porous over time. Small amounts of clear fluid called *edema* may leak out into the surrounding retina. If enough fluid seeps into the macula at the center of the retina, the central vision will become blurry. Macular edema is currently the most common retinal cause of impaired vision in diabetics. Laser treatment directed toward the macula may be able to halt or slow this process.

Proliferative diabetic retinopathy is potentially more serious. The damaged blood vessels start to narrow and eventually close off, resulting in poor circulation to the areas of retina that they feed. As a result, abnormal new blood vessels start to grow from the surface of the retina into the adjacent vitreous gel. These abnormal vessels can either bleed into the vitreous, or form scars that lead to retinal detachments. If detected early enough, these proliferations of abnormal blood vessels can be halted by laser therapy.

For someone with rapidly worsening diabetic retinopathy, it's better to delay cataract surgery until any necessary retinal treatment can be performed and the retinopathy is stabilized. It's also important to have one's blood sugar under control. When the retinopathy is advancing and unstable, especially if the blood sugar control is poor, cataract surgery can actually worsen the blood vessel complications and leakage.

Proceeding with Cataract Surgery

Once the retinopathy has been stabilized, can one proceed with cataract surgery? The surgery can remove the cataract, but it can't reverse vision impairment caused by the diabetic retinopathy. If this impairment is mild, cataract surgery can still provide reasonably good vision. However, if the retinal damage is extensive, the person's vision will still be quite limited even after cataract surgery.

In some cases, the eye doctor may want to remove the cataract because it interferes with the ability to diagnose and treat the diabetic retinopathy. Unfortunately, the surgeon can't know in advance just how much the preexisting retinal disease impairs vision. If you have diabetic retinopathy and a cataract, talk with your ophthalmologist about whether surgery will provide a significant improvement in your vision.

Glaucoma

Since glaucoma and cataracts are very common in older people, it's not surprising that many people have both conditions. Glaucoma is caused by excessive fluid pressure within the eyeball. How does this occur? A clear fluid, the aqueous humor, constantly circulates inside the front of the eyeball. This fluid normally drains through a tiny sieve-like drain at the base of the iris; however, over time this drain can clog, and because the fluid can no longer exit as quickly, an

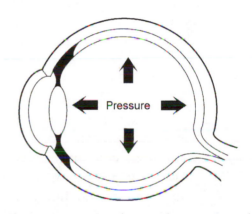

Glaucoma is a condition where impaired aqueous fluid drainage leads to elevated pressure inside the eyeball.

elevated pressure inside the eyeball results. The total amount of fluid is extremely small, only about one-eighth of a teaspoon, so there are no noticeable symptoms and you absolutely can't feel the elevated pressure.

If the fluid pressure is not lowered, it can cause gradual and permanent damage to the optic nerve. Glaucoma is usually treated with eyedrop medications to reduce the eye pressure to a safe level. Sometimes surgery is required.

Can You Have Cataract Surgery?

One of the questions that virtually every glaucoma patient asks is, "Does having glaucoma lower my chances for successful cataract surgery?" Most glaucoma patients who do not have significant vision loss can expect good results from cataract surgery. It is important to realize that any vision loss due to advanced optic nerve damage from glaucoma is permanent and cannot be restored with cataract surgery.

Most people will need to continue their glaucoma drops immediately before and after cataract surgery, but some may be asked to temporarily stop or change a particular glaucoma medication. Patients often are concerned that cataract surgery will aggravate their glaucoma. If you have glaucoma, your eye pressure may vary for a while following cataract surgery, but this is normal and only temporary. Generally, cataract surgery does nothing to worsen glaucoma. In fact, the eye pressure frequently decreases several months after small-incision cataract surgery.

Combining Surgery for Cataracts and Glaucoma

Most people with glaucoma never need glaucoma surgery; however, it is possible that your doctor will determine that in addition to cataract surgery, you also need a surgical procedure called a *trabeculectomy* to keep your glaucoma from progressing. This surgery is done to decrease the risk of damage to the optic nerve by lowering the eye pressure, and it can be done at the same time as cataract surgery.

In a trabeculectomy the surgeon makes a tiny permanent valve-like drain in the eye wall to bypass the clogged natural drainage area. You may wonder what keeps such an incision from scarring and healing shut. To keep the valve open, drugs are applied at the time of surgery that help to prevent the valve from being scarred shut.

Although a trabeculectomy can improve the long-term control of the glaucoma, combining the procedures may delay the recovery of vision from the cataract surgery. Vision may remain blurred for two months or more, especially if eye pressure is initially very low. In addition, there are some risks associated with glaucoma surgery, such as lowering the eye pressure too much.

High Myopia

As explained in an earlier chapter, myopia refers to being nearsighted—you can see things up close without glasses, but you need glasses or contact lenses to see clearly in the distance. Those who become severely nearsighted at an early age are called *high myopes*. Those with myopia have long eyeballs. Just as some people have long feet, some have long eyeballs. The length of the eye is measured from the front, at the cornea, to the back of the eye where the retina is located.

There are two special considerations for cataracts in high myopes. First, cataracts in young myopic patients may be more difficult to diagnose in their earliest stage. And second, these individuals are at a slightly increased risk for retinal detachment occurring several months after surgery.

Diagnosing Early Cataracts in High Myopes

Individuals with long myopic eyes have a tendency to form cataracts at an earlier age, sometimes even in their 40s or 50s. These early myopic cataracts are called *oil droplet cataracts* because they resemble a tiny oil droplet in the center of the lens of the eye. One of the common symptoms of this type of cataract is double vision or seeing ghost images from light sources at night. An example would be seeing several moons in the night sky. As these cataracts progress, they change the optics of the eye such that the myopia actually increases.

The early symptoms of these cataracts may be quite subtle, and their presence may not be entirely obvious during an eye exam. Younger patients are not expected to have cataracts; nor do these cataracts resemble those found in older patients. As a result, these early oil droplet cataracts may escape diagnosis initially.

At first, stronger eyeglass prescriptions can compensate for the increased myopia caused by the cataract. However, as the cataracts get progressively worse, the myopia increases more rapidly and vision even with new glasses, remains poor.

Retinal Detachment in High Myopes

Over the course of their lifetime, individuals with highly myopic eyes are more susceptible to retinal detachment—the sudden separation of the retina from the inner wall of the eyeball. Why? In the longer myopic eye, the sclera and retina are more stretched, which may cause microscopic weak spots in the peripheral retina that are predisposed to tearing. The precipitating factor is the natural aging of the transparent gel-like substance, called the vitreous humor, that occupies the central cavity within our eyeballs and becomes more watery over time. Much like gelatin that has started to liquefy, the more watery the vitreous humor becomes, the more it can slosh around with eye movement.

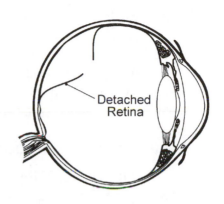

Detached Retina

In an eye with a predisposed weak peripheral retina, this normal sloshing can eventually cause a tear, that in turn leads to a retinal detachment. The latter occurs if enough liquefied vitreous passes through the tear and separates the retina from the back of the eyeball like a sheet of wallpaper. Retinal

The most common type of retinal detachment occurs when there is a tear in the peripheral retina. Vitreous fluid seeps through the break, lifting the thin retina away from the eye wall.

detachments can be surgically repaired, but the vision does not always fully recover.

Although retinal detachments are more likely to occur in highly myopic people than in the rest of the population, the actual odds of this occurring are still very small, less than 5 percent. However, the risk of retinal detachment in predisposed eyes increases slightly during the years following uncomplicated cataract surgery. This is particularly true of young, myopic males. This probably relates to the fact that the artificial lens is much thinner than the natural lens. Cataract surgery therefore creates additional space for the aging vitreous humor to slosh about.

Fortunately, if the cataract is significant, the benefits of surgery still outweigh the risks. People with severe myopia garner one additional benefit from cataract surgery: the power of the IOL selected for them can dramatically improve their distance vision without glasses. When they need cataract surgery in the second eye, some of these patients are actually pleased for this reason. Although patients will likely still need glasses for some tasks, they will have good functional vision for many everyday tasks without glasses for the first time in their lives.

Macular Degeneration

The macula is the small central area of the retina where fine vision and detail are captured. Like other parts of our body, it can become weaker with age. It is estimated that 15 million Americans

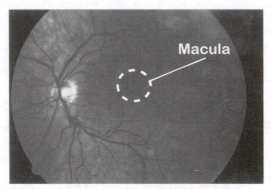

The macula is responsible for fine vision. In the normal eye above, the macula shows up as a dark area in the center of the retina.

have some degree of macular degeneration. This is a general term that covers the entire spectrum of aging change to the macula. Most people will have only milder degrees of macular degeneration and will not experience major vision loss. And, even people with the most severe form of macular degeneration never go completely blind. Although they may lose central vision, they maintain good peripheral vision. Much like age-related hearing loss, vision changes from macular degeneration usually occur very gradually.

A small minority of people with macular degeneration may experience a more rapid decline of their central vision because of a complication called *neovascularization*. This refers to the growth of abnormal blood vessels underneath the weakened macula that eventually start to leak fluid or blood. This permanently damages and scars the macular retinal cells. If these abnormal new blood vessels are discovered, the patient is said to have wet macular degeneration. As long as these abnormal vessels have not formed, the patient is said to have dry macular degeneration.

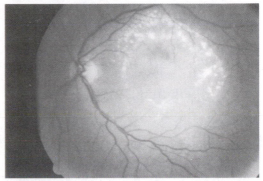

This patient has wet macular degeneration. The whitish areas indicate fluid leakage beneath the macula.

Can You Have Cataract Surgery?

Whether macular degeneration affects one's chances for successful cataract surgery is a matter of some confusion. If the cataract is advanced enough, macular degeneration patients can certainly benefit from having it removed. The surgery should not affect the macular degeneration—the macula is at the back of the eye, and the cataract is closer to the front of the eye. However, how well one sees following cataract surgery depends on the severity of permanent vision loss caused by the macular degeneration. For example, if you have mild macular degeneration and an advanced cataract, you should experience a significant improvement in your vision after surgery. On the other hand, if you have advanced macular degeneration and a mild cataract, you may not see much improvement in your vision at all.

Your doctor will try to determine whether the cataract is significant enough to warrant surgery, although it's impossible to know in advance to what degree your symptoms are caused by the cataract versus the macular degeneration. It isn't possible to test separately the vision loss from the two coexisting conditions. Many people who have both conditions undergo cataract surgery to get whatever partial vision improvement they can. Only then will they have the satisfaction of knowing that they've done everything possible to maximize their vision.

Refractive Surgery

In the previous chapter, we discussed a form of refractive surgery known as LASIK, which improves the ability to see without glasses by reshaping the cornea with a laser. In the 1980s, prior to LASIK, another refractive surgery procedure, *radial keratotomy (RK)*, was the primary method used to treat nearsightedness. Unlike LASIK, RK involved making multiple spoke-like incisions in the cornea to reshape it. Nowadays, RK has been almost completely replaced by LASIK surgery, which achieves better and more stable results. (The RK procedure should not be confused with astigmatic keratotomy, which is an excellent method to treat astigmatism.)

If you have had either of these forms of refractive surgery in the past, you might wonder how the procedure may affect your cataract surgery. You can still have cataract surgery using the same state-of-the-art techniques and IOLs; however, your doctor will must be prepared to deal with a special problem created by the refractive surgery. Since refractive procedures reshape the cornea, it becomes difficult to properly measure the power of the cornea before cataract surgery. The resulting inaccurate measurements make it much harder for the doctor to calculate the appropriate power for the IOL.

If you've had refractive surgery, your ophthalmologist will make the best estimate of the optimum IOL power using a combination of supplemental techniques. The accuracy of these alternative measurements can also be compromised by the presence of the cataract. The farther off the measurements are, the stronger your postoperative glasses will need to be. In some cases, if the IOL power calculation is too far off, it may be necessary to exchange the IOL implant or perhaps to "piggyback" an additional IOL on top of the first one.

Complicated Eyes

A complicated eye refers to one that is more difficult than usual to operate on. It may have certain anatomic features, such as a small pupil, that complicate the steps of the surgery. Or the cataract may have characteristics that make it more challenging to remove, such as with mature brown and mature white cataracts.

> *If you have other eye problems, you can still be a good candidate for cataract surgery especially if the cataract is advanced..*
> —Dr. David Chang

Although a number of factors can make cataract surgery more difficult in some eyes, when you are in experienced hands, the prognosis is still generally excellent.

Small Pupils

For a variety of reasons, a number of patients have pupils that do not dilate very widely after the dilating drops are given. Cataract surgeons refer to these patients as having small pupils. In some individuals the pupil size becomes smaller with age; some individuals with glaucoma have permanently small pupils as a result of having used a glaucoma medicine called *pilocarpine*.

Smaller pupils make intraocular surgery more challenging by providing less working room for the surgeon inside the eye. This increases the chance of tearing the capsular bag, which may require the use of an alternate style of IOL. Fortunately, a surgeon is able to stretch or expand the pupil temporarily, making it easier to remove the cataract and allowing most patients with small pupils to have a good outcome.

Weak Capsular Bag and Zonules

Modern cataract surgery involves preserving the transparent capsular bag that surrounds the eye's lens so that it will permanently support the IOL. Microscopic support ligaments known as *zonules* securely suspend the lens and its capsular bag behind the iris. However, weak or deficient zonules can complicate cataract removal. In addition, the capsular bag itself may be too weak to support the artificial lens implant.

A number of factors increase the chances of having weak zonules or a weak capsular bag. Eye injuries or prior eye surgery such as glaucoma or vitreous surgery can stretch or weaken the support ligaments. People who have an eye condition called *retinopathy of prematurity*, a result of premature birth, often have weak support ligaments. Advanced age may also cause the support ligaments to become fragile.

Another common cause of weak or deficient support ligaments, especially among older Caucasians, is called *exfoliation* or *pseudoexfoliation*. Particularly common among people of Northern European, Russian, or Scandinavian descent, the condition causes microscopic white deposits on the eye's iris and lens that can be seen only with the slit lamp examination.

In many cases, the surgeon has no way of knowing about a weak capsular bag or weak support ligaments before surgery, although a few subtle clinical signs may arouse suspicion. During surgery, the surgeon can tell whether a weakness exists by how the lens behaves during the surgical steps. Once aware of the condition, he or she can use alternative techniques to place the IOL in the eye and still achieve good results.

Mature Brown Cataracts

When certain types of cataracts become very advanced, they become hard and solid, and the central core starts to turn brown. A *mature brown cataract* is more difficult to remove because it takes more ultrasound energy to break it into small pieces for removal. Both the density of the lens and the use of greater ultrasound energy may increase the stresses applied to the capsule and the capsular bag during surgery. This can increase the risk of a tear in the capsular bag. However as discussed earlier, such a complication is manageable.

> *It's difficult to predict exactly how much one's vision will improve after cataract surgery. Other conditions, which may affect vision, must be taken into consideration.*
> —Dr. Howard Gimbel

On rare occasions, the surgeon may decide the cataract's core is too dense to be removed with phacoemulsification and choose to remove the cataract through a large-incision procedure.

Cataract surgery in these advanced cases should still have a good outcome. Since the surgery may take longer, the recovery of vision may be delayed by a few weeks.

Mature White Cataracts

With some advanced cataracts the entire lens turns white. This is the only time that cataracts change the external appearance of the eye. With these cataracts, the normally black pupil also appears white.

Mature white cataracts are more challenging to remove because they make it difficult for the surgeon to see the internal parts of the lens during surgery. The surgeon can use a special dye during the operation to help visualize the necessary lens structures. This type of cataract also carries a slightly higher risk for tearing the capsular bag. In addition, white cataracts make it impossible for the ophthalmologist to examine the back of the eyeball to see if other conditions, such as macular degeneration, might exist. If there are no other abnormalities with the retina or optic nerve, these patients should still achieve a good outcome from cataract surgery.

Pediatric Cataracts

We usually think of cataracts as a condition affecting the elderly. Most parents are surprised and puzzled when their infants are diagnosed with cataracts. Due to genetic or prenatal influences, babies may be born with a cataract affecting one or both eyes, and the density, size, and location can vary considerably. These factors determine whether and how urgently surgery is needed.

Preoperative assessment may involve the child's pediatrician or a geneticist to check for associated disease that may not have been previously diagnosed. *Pediatric ophthalmologists* are specialists in cataract treatment for children.

Treating cataracts in children is much more complex than treating them in adults because the eye tissue changes as it matures. The fact that the immature eye will be changing in size so much in the first few years of life makes the use of intraocular lenses in infants problematic. After age two, IOLs can be used; after this age, moderate, but not extreme, changes in the length of the eye can be anticipated.

If cataract surgery is performed, postoperative care may include contact lens fitting, frequent modifications in the strength of glasses or contact lenses as the eye grows, and eye patching to manage a lazy eye.

In Conclusion

Learning for the first time that you have a cataract, an eye problem that will eventually require surgery, can be a frightening experience. As with any common medical condition, you probably have already heard plenty of piece-meal information from varying sources. Unfortunately, many people worry and delay surgery unnecessarily because of misunderstandings. Our goal in writing this book has been to give you detailed instructions, and to help you understand as much about cataracts and surgery as possible.

The term "medical miracle" is probably overused. However, it is no exaggeration to say that cataract surgery with an artificial lens implant is one of the greatest successes in all of medicine and surgery. As we age, we are repeatedly frustrated to learn that for most natural aging ailments, our only hope is to slow or delay their progression. Fortunately, that is not the case with cataracts. Through this amazing, microsurgical outpatient procedure, we can halt an aging problem that is ruining your eyesight and permanently reverse it.

Cataract surgery is no longer something to avoid or dread. Thanks to modern technology and surgical innovation, the operation and the recovery have become much faster, safer, and easier. The most advanced cataract techniques have eliminated sutures, anesthetic injections, eye bandages, and postoperative restrictions for most patients. Although these more advanced methods require a much greater level of skill and expertise on the part of the surgeon, cataract patients are the clear winners.

Cataract surgery is now the most commonly performed operation in the industrialized world, and millions of North Americans enjoy the benefits of renewed sight every year. The success rate is now among the highest of any operation performed anywhere in the body. Best of all, some people are surprised to find that afterwards they are seeing even better than they ever had before. This is why many of our patients think back upon their cataract surgery as a gift. As eye surgeons, we feel equally blessed. Helping people regain vision they have lost is one of the most gratifying experiences that a physician can have.

We hope that the information we have presented is both informative and reassuring to you. Taking the time to read and learn more about cataracts is a wise investment in your health. Becoming as knowledgeable as possible, having confidence in your surgeon, and having a positive attitude about your condition can help to make your overall surgical experience much easier.

Resources

American Academy of Ophthalmology

Public Information Program
P.O. Box 7424
San Francisco, CA 94120-7424
415-561-8555 Ext. 223
www.eyenet.org

Provides brochures and fact sheets on eye conditions and visual impairment. Web site has a comprehensive database of information about eye diseases and conditions, including up-to-date information on nutrition, treatment, and prevention.

American Council of the Blind

1155 15th Street NW, Suite 1004
Washington, D.C. 20005
800-424-8666
202-467-5081
www.acb.org

A membership organization that advocates for the blind and visually impaired. Offers an information and referral service on all aspects of visual impairment and blindness. Web site includes many resources for the visually impaired, including medical information on macular degeneration, catalogs, books, and related links.

American Foundation for the Blind

11 Penn Plaza, Suite 300
New York, NY 10001
800-232-5463
212-502-7600
212-502-7662 TDD (for hearing impaired)
212-502-7661 (NY residents)
www.afb.org

A national clearinghouse for information about blindness and visual impairment. Offers information for the visually impaired and publishes a *Directory of Services for Blind and Visually Impaired Persons in the U.S. and Canada.* Maintains regional offices. Web site topics include aging and vision loss, education, employment, and technology. Also offers publications and links to other resources.

American Optometric Association

23 Lindbergh Boulevard
St. Louis, MO 63141
314-991-4100
www.theaoa.org

Provides brochures on low vision and other eye problems. Web site answers questions and offers consumer information, tips, and guidelines on eye exams, eye diseases, eye care, and eyewear.

American Society of Cataract and Refractive Surgery (ASCRS)
American Society of Ophthalmic Administrators (ASOA)
4000 Legato Rd. #850
Fairfax, VA 22033
703-591-2220
www.ascrs.org

An organization for ophthalmic surgeons and ophthalmic practice administrators that is a source of education and training programs to advance their skills and expertise. Web site includes a patient-friendly eye care glossary, cataract surgery quiz, "Find A Surgeon" directory, and patient's guide.

Association for Macular Diseases, Inc.
210 East 64th Street
New York, NY 10021
212-605-3719

A national support group that provides members with a newsletter and a phone hotline.

Canadian National Institute for the Blind
www.cnib.ca

Offers a wealth of information and tips for living with low vision, including a handbook for caregivers. Accessible in English or French.

The Center for the Partially Sighted

12301 Wilshire Boulevard, Suite 600
Los Angeles, CA 90025
310-458-3501
www.low-vision.org

Counseling center offering support groups and counseling services for people who are vision impaired. Web site offers information about warning signs and risk factors for vision loss.

Council of Citizens with Low Vision International

800-733-2258
317-254-1332

Serves as an advocacy group for the visually impaired and provides information on low-vision technology. Publishes a newsletter.

Division of Rehabilitation Services

Independent Living Services for Older Individuals Who Are Blind
www.state.sd.us/dhs/drs/il.htm

Federally funded program that offers free services to those age 55 and older who have severe visual impairments. Recipients do not have to be totally blind to qualify. Program requirements vary from state to state. Log on to this Web site or contact your state's division of rehabilitation services for information.

EyeCare America

655 Beach Street
San Francisco, CA 94109-1336
415-447-0381
www.eyecareamerica.org

Public service foundation of the American Academy of Ophthalmology. Free eye exams or glaucoma screenings offered to qualified individuals by member ophthalmologist volunteers. Free educational materials available on eye care. Order materials or request an eye exam by calling one of four helplines listed on the web site.

The Foundation Fighting Blindness

www.blindness.org

An organization that funds research into retinal degenerative disease worldwide. Links to many other sites and organizations. Offers access to up-to-date information about eye diseases.

Lighthouse International

Information and Resource Service
111 East 59th Street
New York, NY 10022-1202
800-829-0500
212-821-9200
E-mail: info@lighthouse.org
www.lighthouse.org

Provides information about vision impairment support groups, locating vision rehabilitation services nationwide, and free publications.

The Macula Foundation

www.macula.org

Sponsored by the Macula Foundation, Inc. and the Association for Macular Diseases. Provides information and support for people with macular degeneration and other macular diseases.

Macular Degeneration Foundation

P.O. Box 9752
San Jose, CA 95157-9752
888-633-3937
408-260-1335
E-mail: eyesight@eyesight.org
www.eyesight.org

Conducts research and educates patients on various aspects of retinal diseases. Web site includes vision care specialists, chat room, books and tapes, research on nutrition, and links to other sites.

Macular Degeneration Help Center

8631 West Third Street, Suite 520E
Los Angeles, CA 90048
888-430-9898
www.amd.org

A coalition of patients, families, and leaders in the fields of vision and aging. Toll-free number has recorded information about age-related macular degeneration, 24 hours a day, 7 days a week. Web site has information about macular degeneration, including the latest news on research and experimental treatments.

Glaucoma Research Foundation

490 Post Street, Street 1427
San Francisco, CA 94102
(800) 826-6693
www.glaucoma.org

The Glaucoma Research Foundation's (GRF) mission is to preserve the sight and independence of individuals with glaucoma. The organization's main focus is public awareness about glaucoma and medical research to find a cure. The site provides information about glaucoma and how it is diagnosed and treated. A newsletter is also available.

National Association for the Visually Handicapped

22 West 21st Street
New York, NY 10010
212-889-3141
E-mail: staff@navh.org
or
3201 Balboa Street
San Francisco, CA 94121
415-221-3201

Health agency that provides assistance to the visually impaired. Web site includes information about services available to people with low vision, plus large-print library-by-mail service, newsletters, and kits of information.

National Eye Institute, National Institutes of Health

2020 Vision Place
Bethesda, MD 20892-3655
301-496-5248
E-mail: 2020@nei.nih.gov

Provides free information to the public about eye disease prevention, treatment, and research. Web site features research results, disease information for patients, clinical studies, low vision resources, and print and audio materials.

National Federation for the Blind

1800 Johnson Street
Baltimore, MD 21230
800-638-7518
410-659-9314
E-mail: nfb@iamdigex.net

Provides referral and job services to the blind and visually impaired, as well as literature in a variety of formats. Web site offers information about services, publications, and resources available to the blind and the vision impaired.

The Pediatric Glaucoma & Cataract Family Association

c/o Alex V. Levin, M.D., FRCSC
The Hospital for Sick Children
Department of Ophthalmology
555 University Ave.
Toronto, Ontario M5G 1X8
416-813-6524
www.pgcfa.org

Support organization for parents of children who have glaucoma or cataracts. The web site provides information on pediatric glaucoma and cataracts via email, online forums, a free e-newsletter, and submitted questions to "Ask the Doc."

Prevent Blindness America

500 E. Remington Road
Schaumberg, IL 60173-4557
800-331-2020 Information hot line
847-843-2020
www.preventblindness.org

Volunteer eye health and safety organization providing public and professional education, community programs, and research aimed at preventing blindness in America. Services include a toll-free information hot line, patient services, and vision screenings. Web site has information on macular degeneration, an Amsler grid, and news about vision issues.

The Women's Eye Health Task Force

Schepens Eye Research Institute
20 Staniford St.
Boston, MA 02114-2500
617-912-0210
www.eri.harvard.edu/wehtf

Task force of the Schepens Eye Research Institute focusing on prevention of blindness in women. Information on lifestyle issues, children's eye exams, eye disease statistics among women, and eye exam checklists, educate women on the gender risk factors of eye disease and how to provide adequate eye care for their families.

Glossary

Anterior capsule: The front of the transparent lens capsular bag, through which an opening must be made surgically in order to remove a cataract and implant an IOL.

Anterior chamber IOL: IOL designed for implantation in front of the iris.

Accommodating IOL: Type of IOL designed to move within the eye in order to provide partial focusing ability.

Capsular bag: The transparent membrane surrounding the entire lens of the eyeball.

Cataract: Loss of transparency of the natural lens.

Combined procedure: Two separate operations being performed at the same sitting. In the context of cataracts, this usually refers to glaucoma surgery being performed coincident with cataract surgery.

Conjunctiva: Thin, transparent mucous membrane that overlies the white sclera, and lines the inner aspect of the upper and lower lids.

Conjunctivitis: Inflammation of the conjunctiva. While this is a general term, it is often used in reference to an external eye infection.

Complicated eye: In the context of cataract surgery, this term refers to an eye that has anatomical features that make surgery more difficult.

Cornea: Transparent, dome-shaped structure at the front of the eyeball through which all light rays enter the eye interior.

Glossary

Corneal clouding: Vision-impairing loss of corneal transparency. Depending upon the underlying cause and severity, this condition may be temporary or permanent.

Cortical cataract: Type of cataract where the haze is predominantly in the regions closest to the front and rear of the lens.

Diabetic retinopathy: Progressive retinal disorder that results from diabetes and the associated circulatory abnormalities.

Diffuse cataract: Refers to a cataract where the entire lens is uniformly hazy.

Dilating drops: Medications administered by eyedrops in order to temporarily expand the pupil. Used to permit visualization of the interior eye for either examination or surgery.

Diopter: Standard optical unit of measure. In the context of eyes, this is the unit for measuring refractive error or the power of prescription eyeglasses.

Dry eye: Clinical term describing a relative lack of surface tear lubrication that typically results in symptoms of minor discomfort.

Dry macular degeneration: See macular degeneration.

Exfoliation (psuedoexfoliation): Non-symptomatic eye condition characterized by microscopic changes visible during a dilated eye examination. Often associated with increased difficulty in performing cataract surgery, due either to poor pupil dilation or weakness to the capsular bag support.

Extracapsular surgery: Type of cataract surgery in which the capsular bag supporting the original lens is preserved in order to hold the IOL.

Floater: Moving shadows in the field of vision. The usual cause is age-related liquefaction and clumping of the vitreous gel within the central ocular cavity.

Focal cataract: Refers to a cataract in which only portions of the lens are hazy

Foldable IOL: IOL made of silicone or acrylic plastic to allow it to be folded for insertion through a small cataract incision.

Free radical: Chemical molecules implicated in damage to tissue. They may be caused by UV light.

General anesthesia: Type of anesthesia where the patient is unconscious and a breathing tube connected to a respirator is used.

Glaucoma: Eye disease characterized by progressive damage to the optic nerve. The usual cause is prolonged, abnormal elevation of the intraocular fluid pressure, which is treatable with medication or surgery.

Halo: Symptom of rings appearing around point sources of light. Typically noticeable at night.

Haptic: Flexible, wire-like support member of the intraocular lens. The two haptics center the lens implant within the capsular support bag.

High myopia: Higher than average degree of myopia associated with an elongated eyeball.

Hyperopia: Refractive error in which light rays are misfocused behind, rather than on the retina. Called farsightedness because closer objects appear more blurred than distant objects.

Intracapsular surgery: Cataract surgery in which the capsular bag is removed together with the lens. This is an older technique of surgery that is not currently used.

Intraocular lens (IOL): Artificial lens permanently implanted in the eye.

Intraocular pressure: Internal fluid pressure of the eyeball. Prolonged elevation can lead to glaucoma.

Iris: Colored structure located behind the cornea that functions like a curtain to regulate the amount of light that passes to the back of the eye.

LASIK (Laser in situ keratomileusis): Refractive operation that involves laser-guided reshaping of the cornea beneath a thin, surgically created flap.

Lens: Transparent intraocular tissue, located behind the pupil, that helps bring rays of light to a focus on the retina.

Lidocaine: A common injectable anesthetic drug.

Macula: Circular central-most region of the retina, which produces detailed, fine central vision.

Macular degeneration: Age related deterioration of the macula, which impairs the central vision. If abnormal vessels grow and leak fluid beneath the weakened macula, the condition is called "wet." If this has not occurred, the condition is called "dry."

Macular edema: Clear fluid collecting in the macula, which impairs central vision. The fluid source is abnormally porous capillaries in the retina.

Mature brown cataract: Extremely advanced cataract stage in which the central nucleus becomes extremely solid.

Mature white cataract: Extremely advanced cataract stage in which the lens turns white and becomes totally opaque.

Monofocal IOL: Type of IOL that provides optimal focus without glasses at a single distance.

Monovision: Vision in which two eyes each see at different distances without glasses. If achieved through contact lenses or IOLs, typically one eye sees better at a distance without glasses, and the second eye is focused closer without glasses.

Multifocal IOL: Type of IOL that provides optimal focus without glasses at more than one distance.

Myopia: Refractive error in which light rays are misfocused in front of, rather than on the retina. Called nearsightedness because without glasses, the patient sees clearer up close, but is blurry in the distance.

Non-proliferative diabetic retinopathy: a form of retinopathy characterized by leaky, porous blood vessels.

Nuclear cataract: Type of cataract where the haze is predominantly in the centermost region of lens.

Oil droplet cataract: Type of nuclear cataract most often seen in young myopes, and so-named because it looks like an oil droplet to the examining eye specialist.

Optic nerve: Nerve that transmits vision from the retina to the brain.

Optician: Eye professional who is licensed to fit and dispense eyeglasses and sometimes contacts.

Optometrist: Doctor of optometry (OD) specializing in vision problems, treating vision conditions with spectacles, contact lenses, low vision aids and vision therapy, and prescribing medications for certain eye diseases.

Ophthalmologist: Eye physician who is a medical doctor and who specializes in medical and surgical treatment of the eye. General ophthalmologists do not sub-specialize and perform the majority of cataract surgeries. Specialist ophthalmologists sub-specialize in treatment of certain disorders such as those of the retina or cornea.

Pediatric cataract: Cataract that develops in an infant or child.

Phacoemulsification (Phaco): Surgical technique in which the cataract is ultrasonically fragmented and aspirated.

Pilocarpine: Glaucoma eyedrop medication that also constricts the pupil.

Pledget: Small thin sponge that can placed just beneath the eyelid to administer eye medications.

Posterior capsule: The back part of the transparent lens capsular bag, which is preserved in extracapsular cataract surgery in order to support the IOL.

Posterior chamber IOL: an IOL designed for implantation behind the iris.

Presbyopia: Normal age-induced refractive error characterized by the inability to focus. up close despite clear distant vision. Occurs after the age of 40 due to the normal loss of lens flexibility.

Proliferative diabetic retinopathy: Form of retinopathy marked by abnormal, new blood **vessels** grow from the retina into the vitreous. These vessels can bleed or scar, leading to retinal detachment.

Pupil: Circular opening in the iris through which light passes in order to enter the back of the eye.

Radial keratotomy: Refractive surgical procedure for myopia using radial cuts in the cornea.

Refractive error: Optical imperfection in an otherwise healthy eye that results in blurred vision without glasses at certain distances.

Regional anesthesia: Type of local anesthesia in which anesthetic is injected in the eye region.

Retina: The thin, light-sensitive tissue that lines the back half of the eyeball and captures and registers vision.

Retinal detachment: Condition in which the retina separates from the inner eye wall.

Retinopathy of prematurity: Retinal condition associated with premature birth, which carries a higher risk of retinal detachment.

Sclera: White wall of the eyeball.

Secondary cataract: the clouding of the back of the posterior capsule months or years after cataract surgery. Accurately called a secondary membrane, the term is misleading since cataracts never recur.

Secondary IOL: An IOL that is inserted during a separate operation subsequent to the original cataract surgery.

Secondary membrane: Condition in which the posterior capsule becomes cloudy. months to years following successful cataract surgery.

Small pupils: Refers to eyes in which the pupil does not dilate normally following insertion of dilating drops.

Snellen chart: Standard eye chart for testing distance vision.

Specialist ophthalmologist: See ophthalmologist.

Speculum: Device that holds open the eyelids during eye surgery.

Stye: Infected oil gland occurring in the edge of the eyelid.

Subcapsular cataract: Type of cataract where the haze is located adjacent to the anterior front) or posterior (rear) lens capsule.

Tear duct: Microscopic drainage channel for tears located in the corner of the upper and lower lid closest to the nose.

Tonometer: Instrument used to measure the internal eye fluid pressure

Topical anesthesia: Anesthesia administered via eyedrop installation. Applications range from eye examinations to cataract surgery.

Toric IOL: A special IOL that is designed to reduce higher degrees of pre-existing astigmatism.

Trabeculectomy: Surgical procedure for glaucoma, in which a valve-like channel for fluid drainage is created in the eye wall.

20/20 vision: Ability to read the rows on the eye chart that correlate with "normal" visual acuity.

20/15 vision: Ability to read the row smaller than the 20/20 row on the eye chart. This is closer to "perfect" visual acuity.

Uveitis (Iritis): Inflammation occurring within the interior of the eye.

Visual acuity: Refers to the quality of central vision.

Vitreous humor: Semi-solid, gel-like material that fills the central cavity of the eyeball.

Wet macular degeneration: See macular degeneration.

YAG capsulotomy: Non-surgical, vision-restoring treatment for a secondary membrane.

Zonules: The microscopic ligaments that support the lens and capsular bag.

Index

20/20 vision, 20, 21

A

accommodating intraocular lens, 30, 31, 70
accommodation, 3, 6, 30
after cataract
    see secondary membrane
age
    as a risk factor, 13
age-related cataract, 9, 12, 13
allergies, 20
alpha-crystallins, 13
American Academy of Ophthalmology, 8
anatomy
    of the eye, 1–4, 40, 75
anterior chamber, 2
anterior chamber intraocular lens, 32
antibiotic eyedrops, 60
antioxidants, 15
aphakia, 25
aphakic
    contact lenses, 26, 27, 75
    glasses, 25–27, 75
aqueous humor, 2, 81

artificial tears, 60
aspirin, 47
asthma, 14, 20, 48
astigmatic keratotomy, 70–72
astigmatism, 6, 42, 43, 62
    astigmatic keratotomy, 70–72
    multifocal intraocular lens, 69

B

bacteria, 44
benefits of surgery, 52
bifocals, 63
blindness, 7, 8, 13
    see also aphakia
blinking, 4
blood sugar, 7, 14, 16
    diabetic retinopathy, 78, 80
blood thinners, 47
blood vessel growth, 87
blurry vision, 7, 10, 56, 65
    after cataract surgery, 56–58
board certification, 38

C

camera, 1, 3, 4
capsular bag, 3, 41, 43, 64–67
    tearing, 91, 92

after cataract surgery, 53, 56, 57

diopters, 38

double images, 10, 84

drifting shadows
  see floaters

driving
  after cataract surgery, 62

driving test, 36

dry eyes, 23, 60, 75

E

edema, 79

emphysema, 14, 20

examination, 18–24

exfoliation, 90

extracapsular surgery, 40
  types, 40–43

eye
  anatomy, 1–4, 40, 75
  care specialists, 16, 17
  colored discharge after surgery, 54
  diseases, 14
  disorders, 6, 78-93
  examination, 18–24
  exterior, 22, 23
  interior, 23, 24
  history, 19
  lubrications, 4
  pressure, 7
    see also glaucoma
    measuring, 24
  proteins, 13
  redness, 56
  scratchy, 56

trauma, 15

eye care specialists, 17, 18

eye color
  see iris

eye disorders, 6, 78–93

eye pressure
  drainage, 81

eyedrops
  anti-inflammatory, 59, 60
  antibiotic, 44
  dilating, 49
  insertion, 44–47
  topical anesthesia, 47–50

eyeglass prescription, 11, 19, 37, 42
  after cataract surgery, 52, 62

eyeglasses
  after cataract surgery, 61, 62
  reducing dependence, 68–77

eyelid, 22

F

family history, 13, 14

farsightedness, 31

finding cataract surgeon, 37, 38

flexible lens
  see intraocular lens (IOL)

floaters, 4, 56, 67

fluid pressure, 19, 67
  see also glaucoma

focal cataract, 23

focal zones, 69

focus
  see accommodation

foldable intraocular lens
  see intraocular lens (IOL)

Food and Drug Administration
  (FDA), 29-31, 34, 40, 73
free radicals, 13

G

general anesthesia, 49, 53
general ophthalmologist, 17, 37
ghost images, 11, 69, 84
glare, 10
  secondary, 65
glaucoma, 7, 19, 24, 81–83
  with cataract surgery, 82
  eyedrops, 82

H

halos, 56, 57, 69, 70
heart disease, 20
high myopia, 78, 83–86
  diagnosing, 84
hyperopic, 31
  see also farsightedness
hypertension, 20

I

infection, 53
insurance, 31, 34, 37, 77
intracapsular surgery, 41
intraocular lens (IOL), 25–34
  accommodating, 30, 31
  anterior chamber, 32
  characteristics, 28
  composition, 31, 32
  history, 27, 28
  implant power, 38–40
  microscopic movement, 58
  monofocal, 29
  multifocal, 29, 30

placement, 32
posterior chamber, 32
secondary, 31
testing standards, 74
toric, 30
types, 29–31
intraocular pressure, 24, 51, 53
  see also glaucoma
intravenous (IV) line, 48
IOL
  see intraocular lens (IOL)
IOL Master, 40
iris, 2, 53
  drain, 81
  examination, 24
  scarring, 76
iritis, 14

L

large-incision cataract surgery,
  40, 42, 43, 91
laser, 66, 77
laser in situ keratomileusis
  see LASIK surgery
LASIK surgery, 76, 77, 88
  with cataract surgery, 77
lazy eye, 92
lens, 2, 3, 40
  examination, 24
  removal, 35-43, 44-54
lens implant power, 38–40
light sensitivity, 56, 60
local anesthesia, 42

M

macula, 86

About the Authors

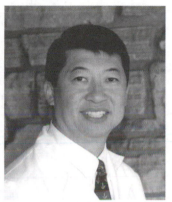

David F. Chang, M.D., is an ophthalmologist in private practice in Los Altos, where he has practiced since 1984. He is one of only a few ophthalmologists in Northern California to limit his practice to cataract surgery. "Helping people regain vision they have lost is one of the most gratifying experiences that a physician can have. Having steered thousands of patients through this experience, I have an appreciation for a patient's most common concerns and fears."

Dr. Chang graduated Phi Beta Kappa and *summa cum laude* from Harvard College and earned his Medical Degree from Harvard Medical School. He completed his ophthalmology residency at the University of California, San Francisco, where he is now Clinical Professor of Ophthalmology teaching cataract surgery to ophthalmologists in training.

As an internationally acclaimed cataract expert, Dr. Chang regularly lectures on cataract techniques to other surgeons in the U.S. and abroad. Among his awards are the UCSF Teaching Award (1995), the Transamerica Lecture (University of California, San Francisco 2001), the Wolfe Lecture (University of Iowa 2002), the Gold Medal from the India Intraocular Implant and Refractive Society (Chennai 2003), and the American Academy of Ophthalmology Honor Award (2002) and Secretariat Award (2003).

Dr. Chang has been an associate examiner for the American Board of Ophthalmology, which confers board certification. He serves on a national advisory panel for the board re-certification examination in cataract surgery. He has authored numerous papers and chapters on cataract surgery, and has written a textbook on advanced cataract surgical techniques. He is on the editorial board of several ophthalmology journals and publications, and is Co-Chief Medical Editor for *Cataract & Refractive Surgery Today.*

In 2002, Dr. Chang was named the Chairman of the Cataract Program Sub-committee for the American Academy of Ophthalmology Annual Meeting. This is the largest and most prestigious ophthalmology meeting in the world. He organized and co-chaired the first three American Academy of Ophthalmology *Spotlight on Cataracts* Symposia. He was also selected to be the cataract editor for two online educational sites: the *American Academy of Ophthalmology*'s "Specialty Updates," and the *Ocular Surgery News* cyber-text "Ophthalmic Hyperguides."

Dr. Chang is a consultant for several ophthalmic research companies, and will be heading U.S. clinical trials on the Visiogen accommodating IOL. He has achieved several local firsts in cataract surgery. He was the first surgeon in the Bay Area to implant the toric IOL for astigmatism, and the first in Northern California to implant the multifocal IOL, the implantable miniature telescope, and the artificial iris implant. Dr. Chang is in the current national edition of *Best Doctors in America* and is listed in the current "Best Doctors" surveys in *Bay Area Consumers Checkbook, San Francisco Magazine,* and *San Jose Magazine.*

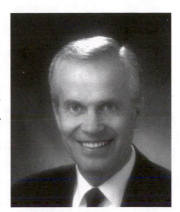

Howard Gimbel, M.D. MPH, is the Founder, Medical Director, and Senior Surgeon of the Gimbel Eye Centres in Calgary and Edmonton, Alberta, Canada. Since February 2000, he has also been Professor and Chairman, Department of Ophthalmology, Loma Linda University School of Medicine, Loma Linda, California, USA. Through his commitment to ophthalmology, he has personally restored or enhanced the vision of more than 75,000 eyes. "I'm grateful for having the privilege to be God's instrument to enhance the vision of so many people."

Dr. Gimbel received his Doctor of Medicine (1960) and Master of Public Health (1978) from Loma Linda University in California. He completed his internship and ophthalmology residency at the White Memorial Medical Center in Los Angeles. In 1964, Dr. Gimbel began practicing as an eye specialist in Calgary. His fascination with equipment compelled Dr. Gimbel to acquire an ever-growing collection of new instruments to diagnose and treat eye disorders. He became the first surgeon in Canada to use an ultrasonic probe to remove cataracts by phacoemulsification, and the first to use an Nd:YAG laser to open secondary membrane cataracts and perform other delicate internal eye procedures. The Calgary Centre was the first institution in Canada to use an Excimer Laser to do refractive corneal surgery in June of 1990.

Research is also an important aspect of practice in a private as well as an academic practice. Dr. Gimbel and his associates are contributing to the body of knowledge in the world of ophthalmology through clinical research programs on cataract and refractive surgery, glaucoma, anterior segment surgery, and prevention of eye disease.

Surgeons from around the world have studied the innovative techniques Dr. Gimbel has developed. Dr. Gimbel also broadcasts live surgeries by satellite to large groups of doctors attending international meetings in North and South America, Europe, and Japan. He has produced numerous videos and articles for peer-reviewed journals and professional magazines, as well as written books and contributed chapters to several medical books. In addition, a fellowship program at Gimbel Eye Centre trains two doctors a year in clinical, research, and surgical aspects of cataract and refractive ophthalmology.

In 1992, Dr. Gimbel received the Alberta Order of Excellence for his ability to combine technical excellence with the art of caring in an atmosphere of open communication. He was commended for using innovation to raise the standards of medical care in Alberta, and for his global influence as an educator at the forefront of microsurgical developments. In 1996 his peers voted him one of the top ophthalmologists in the world.

Dr. Gimbel has been a guest speaker at numerous universities, eye institutes, and eye society meetings around the world. He is on faculty at the University of Calgary, the University of California at San Francisco, and Loma Linda University where he currently is the Chair of the Department of Ophthalmology.

Also from Addicus Books

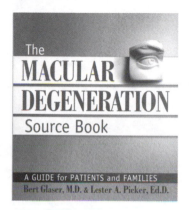

The Macular Degeneration Source Book
A Guide for Patients and Families

Bert Glaser, M.D and Lester A. Picker, Ed.D.

Author Bert Glaser, M.D., is a retinal specialist who has treated thousands of patients with macular degeneration. In the *Macular Degeneration Source Book* he answers questions to commonly asked questions, including treatment options. 155 pages.

$14.95

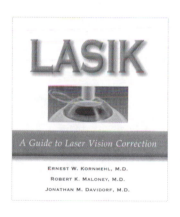

LASIK : A Guide to Laser Vision Correction

Ernest W. Kornmehl, M.D., Robert K. Maloney, M.D., Jonathan M. Davidorf, M.D.

LASIK—the laser vision correction surgery has become one of the most popular vision correction surgeries in the nation. More than 2 million procedures are being performed annually.

But, before you entrust your eyes to a surgeon, make sure you become an informed consumer. In *LASIK—A Guide to Laser Vision Correction,* three respected ophthalmologists help you understand the benefits and risks of the surgery. 130 pages.

$14.95

Other Consumer Health Titles from Addicus Books
Visit our online catalog at www.AddicusBooks.com

Please send:

_____copies of_____
(Title of book)

at $_____each   TOTAL: _____

Nebraska residents add 5% sales tax   _____

Shipping/Handling
  $4.00 postage for first book.
  $1.10 postage for each additional book   _____

  TOTAL ENCLOSED: _____

Name _____

Address _____

City_____State_____Zip _____

☐ **Visa**   ☐ **MasterCard**   ☐ **American Express**

Credit card number _____Expiration date _____

Order by credit card, personal check or money order. Send to:

Addicus Books
Mail Order Dept.
P.O. Box 45327
Omaha, NE 68145
Or, order **TOLL FREE: 800-352-2873**
or online at
www.AddicusBooks.com